615 Rus
RUS Ant
side effects

DISCARD

WELLINGTON MEDIA CENTRE

Antidepressants and Their Side Effects

Managing the Risks

ANTIDEPRESSANTS

Antidepressants and Advertising: Marketing Happiness

Antidepressants and Psychology: Talk Therapy vs. Medication

Antidepressants and Social Anxiety: A Pill for Shyness?

Antidepressants and Suicide: When Treatment Kills

Antidepressants and the Critics: Cure-Alls or Unnatural Poisons?

Antidepressants and the Pharmaceutical Companies:
Corporate Responsibilities

Antidepressants and Their Side Effects: Managing the Risks

The Development of Antidepressants: The Chemistry of Depression

The Future of Antidepressants: The New Wave of Research

The History of Depression: The Mind-Body Connection

"Natural" Alternatives to Antidepressants:
St. John's Wort, Kava Kava, and Others

Prozac: North American Culture and the Wonder Drug

Psychostimulants as Antidepressants: Worth the Risk?

ANTIDEPRESSANTS

Antidepressants and Their Side Effects

Managing the Risks

by Craig Russell

Mason Crest Publishers

Philadelphia

Mason Crest Publishers Inc.
370 Reed Road
Broomall, Pennsylvania 19008
(866) MCP-BOOK (toll free)

Copyright © 2007 by Mason Crest Publishers. All rights reserved. No part of this publication may be reproduced or transmitted in any form or by any means, electronic or mechanical, including photocopying, recording, taping, or any information storage and retrieval system, without permission from the publisher.

First printing
1 2 3 4 5 6 7 8 9 10

Library of Congress Cataloging-in-Publication Data

Russell, Craig, 1952–
  Antidepressants and their side effects : managing the risks / by Craig Russell.
     p. cm. — (Antidepressants)
  Includes bibliographical references and index.
  ISBN 1-4222-0097-3   ISBN 1-4222-0094-9 (series)
  1. Antidepressants—Juvenile literature. 2. Antidepressants—Side effects—Juvenile literature. I. Title. II. Series.
  RM332.R87 2006
  615'.78—dc22
                                2006004321

Interior design by MK Bassett-Harvey.
Interiors produced by Harding House Publishing Service, Inc.
www.hardinghousepages.com.
Cover design by Peter Culatta.
Printed in the Hashemite Kingdom of Jordan.

This book is meant to educate and should not be used as an alternative to appropriate medical care. Its creators have made every effort to ensure that the information presented is accurate—but it is not intended to substitute for the help and services of trained professionals.

Contents

Introduction 6

1. Antidepressants and Side Effects 9

2. Weighing Risks and Benefits 25

3. Antidepressants and Violence: Fact or Excuse? 43

4. Coping With Side Effects 59

5. Withdrawal 77

6. Lawsuits 91

Further Reading 100

For More Information 101

Glossary 102

Bibliography 103

Index 109

Picture Credits 111

Biographies 112

Introduction
by Andrew M. Kleiman, M.D.

From ancient Greece through the twenty-first century, the experience of sadness and depression is one of the many that define humanity. As long as human beings have felt emotions, they have endured depression. Experienced by people from every race, socioeconomic class, age group, and culture, depression is an emotional and physical experience that millions of people suffer each day. Despite being described in literature and music; examined by countless scientists, philosophers, and thinkers; and studied and treated for centuries, depression continues to remain as complex and mysterious as ever.

In today's Western culture, hearing about depression and treatments for depression is common. Adolescents in particular are bombarded with information, warnings, recommendations, and suggestions. It is critical that adolescents and young people have an understanding of depression and its impact on an individual's psychological and physical health, as well as the treatment options available to help those who suffer from depression.

Why? Because depression can lead to poor school performance, isolation from family and friends, alcohol and drug abuse, and even suicide. This doesn't have to be the case, since many useful and promising treatments exist to relieve the suffering of those with depression. Treatments for depression may also pose certain risks, however.

Since the beginning of civilization, people have been trying to alleviate the suffering of those with depression. Modern-day medicine and psychology have taken the understanding and treatment of depression to new heights. Despite their shortcomings, these treatments have helped millions and millions of people lead happier, more fulfilling and prosperous lives that would not be possible in generations past. These treatments, however, have their own risks, and for some people, may not be effective at all. Much work in neuroscience, medicine, and psychology needs to be done in the years to come.

Many adolescents experience depression, and this book series will help young people to recognize depression both in themselves and in those around them. It will give them the basic understanding of the history of depression and the various treatments that have been used to combat depression over the years. The books will also provide a basic scientific understanding of depression, and the many biological, psychological, and alternative treatments available to someone suffering from depression today.

Each person's brain and biology, life experiences, thoughts, and day-to-day situations are unique. Similarly, each individual experiences depression and sadness in a unique way. Each adolescent suffering from depression thus requires a distinct, individual treatment plan that best suits his or her needs. This series promises to be a vital resource for helping young people recognize and understand depression, and make informed and thoughtful decisions regarding treatment.

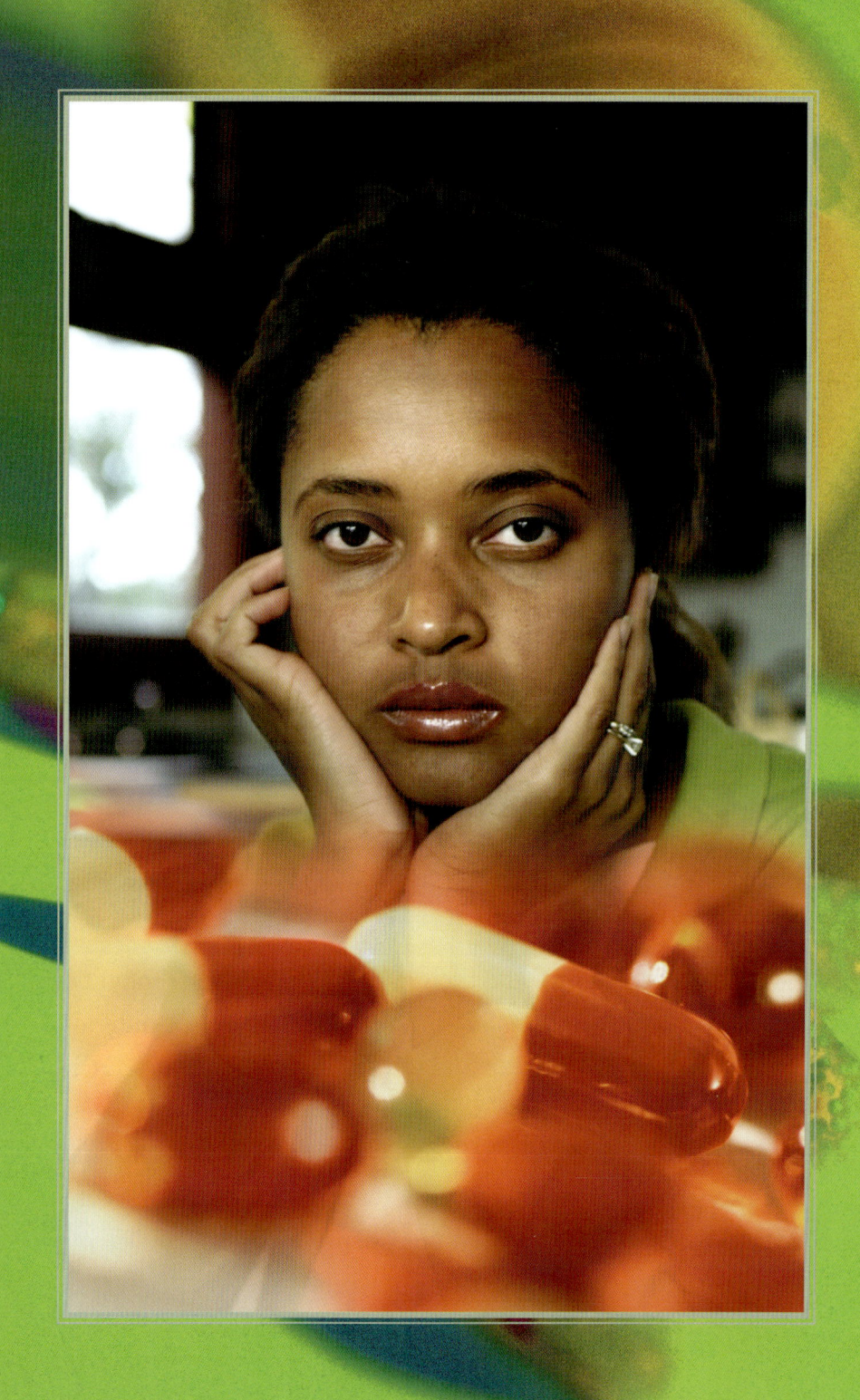

Chapter 1

Antidepressants and Side Effects

Most people would think that Brooke Shields had it all: beauty, wealth, fame. She became a model when she was just eleven months old, and by fifteen, she was a movie star. But in 2003, shortly after giving birth to her first child, she found herself staring out the window of her Manhattan apartment and thinking about killing herself.

"I really didn't want to live anymore," she said. She started having feelings of self-doubt and imagined her daughter flying through the air before hitting a wall and sliding down it.

She was suffering from **postpartum depression**, which affects about one of every ten American mothers. Luckily, the treatment for this is very effective, according to Dr. Donnica Moore, the president of Sapphire Women's Health in Far Hills, New Jersey. It usually consists of a combination of therapy and medication, as well as rest and help from friends and family.

"Without therapy, I wouldn't have understood as much," Shields said, "and I think that without medicine, I would not have been clear enough." She adds, however, that the drug did have a few side effects. "It made my tongue [throb]," she said. "I sounded like I was drunk all the time. [And then] it was devastating when I went off of it because I went off of it cold turkey, which was a huge mistake."

The medicine she took was Paxil® (paroxetine), which is one of a family of antidepressants called selective serotonin reuptake inhibitors, or SSRIs. These SSRIs have become the most commonly prescribed type of antidepressant drugs in the United States. Besides Paxil, this group includes Prozac® (fluoxetine), Zoloft® (sertraline), Luvox® (fluvoxamine),

Brand Names vs. Generic Names

Talking about psychiatric drugs can be confusing, because every drug has at least two names: its "generic name" and the "brand name" that the pharmaceutical company uses to market the drug. Generic names come from the drugs' chemical structure, while drug companies use brand names to inspire public recognition and loyalty for their products.

Antidepressants and Side Effects 11

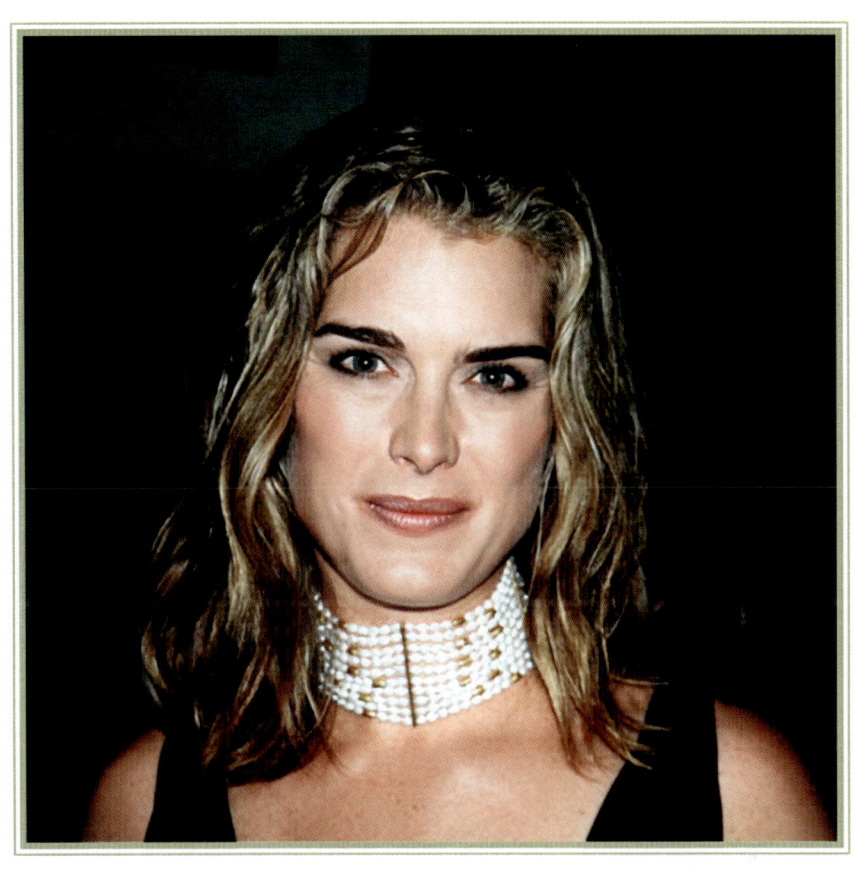

An antidepressant helped Brooke Shields successfully battle postpartum depression.

Celexa® (citalopram), and Lexapro® (escitalopram). Between 2000 and 2004, the number of prescriptions written for antidepressants in the United States increased from 98 million to 146.5 million, making SSRIs the second most prescribed type of medication in the country (the most prescribed is ***codeine***). One in ten American women take an antidepressant, and antidepressants' use is increasing among children and teenagers as well. Antidepressants have become a multi-billion-dollar industry.

What Is Depression?

As their name implies, antidepressants are used to treat depression, which is one of the most common mental disorders in the United States. Depression is more than just feeling unhappy; it goes much deeper and lasts much longer. The *American Heritage Dictionary* defines depression as "a psychiatric disorder characterized by an inability to concentrate, insomnia, loss of appetite, **anhedonia**, feelings of extreme sadness, guilt, helplessness and hopelessness, and thoughts of death." About twenty million Americans suffer from some form of depression every year, and as much as one-quarter of the population will become depressed at some point in their lives. Women are twice as likely as men to be diagnosed with depression.

Serotonin

Besides being found in the human brain, serotonin is also found in such things as human blood, wasp stings, scorpion venom, pineapples, bananas, and various nuts. Adult humans have about 5–10 mg of serotonin in their bodies. Ninety percent is in the intestines, while the other 10 percent is found in blood platelets and in the brain. Doctors believe serotonin plays a role in disorders such as schizophrenia and depression.

How Do Antidepressants Work?

Antidepressants apparently work by changing the chemistry of the brain, which contains billions of specialized cells called neurons. It's these neurons that allow a person to learn, to think, and to remember. Whenever a person feels or thinks

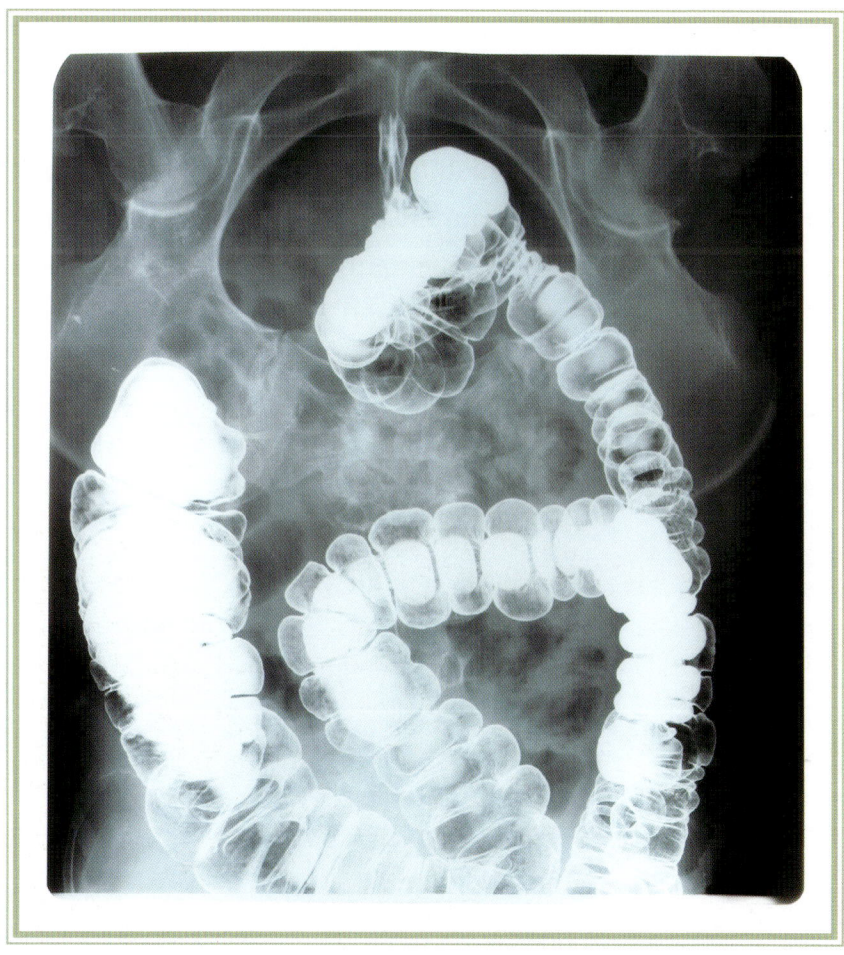

Although most people connect serotonin with brain function, 90 percent of the body's serotonin is found in the intestines.

anything, millions of neurons are communicating with one another.

Neurotransmitters allow this communication to take place. This word's prefix, *neuro-*, refers to nerves and the nervous system, while a "transmitter" is a device that sends information from one place to another. A television remote control is one example of a transmitter.

Neurotransmitters are chemicals that send information across the junction, or synapse, between one nerve cell and another, or between a nerve cell and a muscle. The body stores them in axons, which are found at the end of nerve cells. When an electrical impulse traveling along the nerve reaches the axon, it releases the neurotransmitter, which then

Aspirin

Aspirin is the most popular drug in the world. People take 50 billion aspirin tablets every year. It's also one of the cheapest. Generic brands of aspirin cost about one cent per tablet. Aspirin's scientific name is acetylsalicylic acid, which is based on salicylic acid. It was originally extracted from the bark of the white willow tree. The Haudenosaunee, or Iroquois, of New York State used ground white willow bark in a tea to relieve headaches, fever, sore muscles, chills, rheumatism, and general aches and pains.

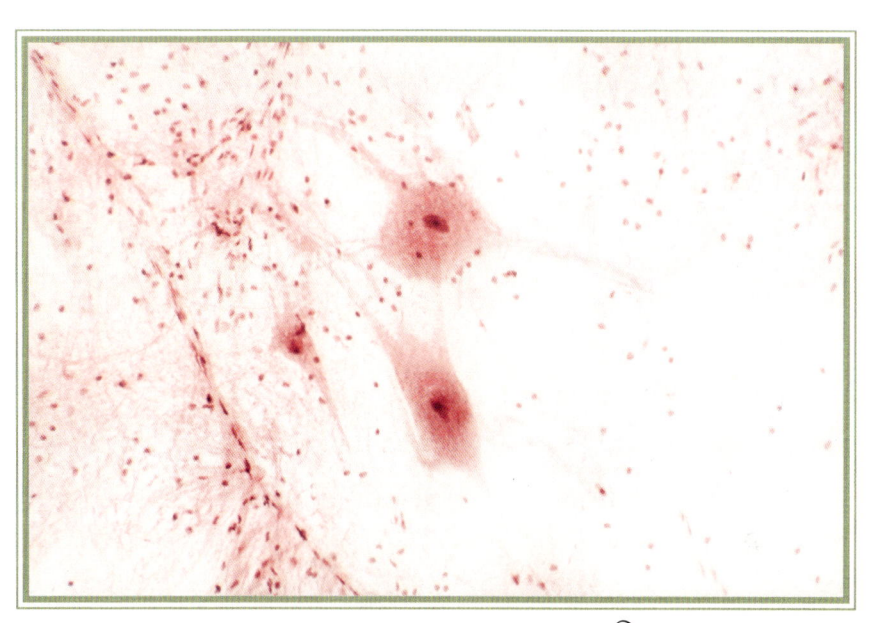

An image of nerve cells, magnified hundreds of times, shows the cells' spiky dendrites, as well as the nuclei at their centers. Neurotransmitters carry electrical impulses across the spaces between these cells.

moves across the synapse. Some neurotransmitters increase that impulse, while others decrease it. Scientists have identified approximately 300 neurotransmitters in the human body.

One of these neurotransmitters is called serotonin. The amount of serotonin in a person's body affects mood, emotion, sleep, and appetite. Antidepressants apparently make it harder for the body to absorb its natural production of serotonin, thereby changing the brain's chemistry. However, scientists are still not sure exactly how these medications work.

16   Antidepressants and Their Side Effects

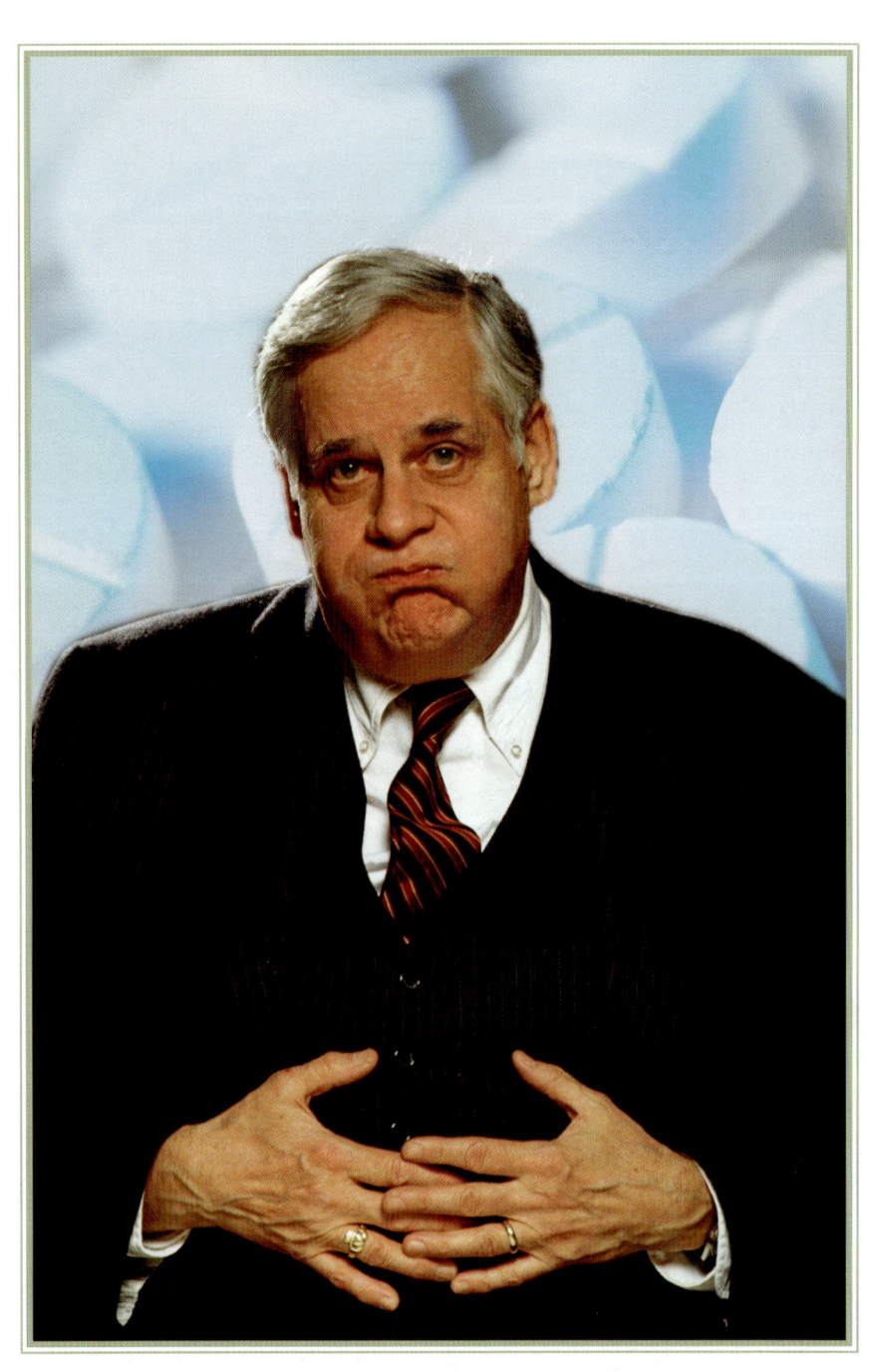

One of aspirin's unwanted side effects may be an upset stomach.

What Is a Side Effect?

Unfortunately, this success often has a price in the form of side effects. A side effect is an unwanted effect that goes hand-in-hand with the main effect. One of aspirin's main effects, for instance, is to relieve pain. However, aspirin often causes stomach bleeding. In relieving that pain, the aspirin might also upset your stomach. An upset stomach, then, is a side effect of aspirin. It's not wanted, but it goes along with relieving pain. You may not be able to have one without the other.

Antidepressants' Side Effects

Side effects have plagued antidepressants ever since they were discovered in the 1950s. The first antidepressant, iproniazid, for

Tricyclics

Tricyclics were among the first antidepressants, coming to the marketplace in the 1960s. Their name comes from the three-ring chemical structure of their molecules. Tricyclic antidepressants include Elavil® (amitriptyline), Tofranil® (imipramine), and Surmontil® (trimipramine). For more than twenty years, tricyclics were the main drug prescribed for people with depression. In some ways, these drugs work like SSRIs by affecting the production and reabsorption of neurotransmitters. Unlike SSRIs, however, they are less selective about which neurotransmitters they affect, and as a result, have more potential side effects than SSRIs.

example, was developed as a drug for tuberculosis, but doctors found that it also helped improve the mood of the patients taking it; unfortunately, they also found that patients who took iproniazid and then ate cheese or drank wine sometimes died. Substances in the cheese or wine combined with substances in the iproniazid to cause problems in the body's cardiovascular system, including severe high blood pressure and hemorrhages. Iproniazid was also suspected of causing **jaundice** and was pulled from the market. This led to a search for a better drug.

The second antidepressant was called imipramine. It was first of a group of drugs called tricyclics. But this drug, too, had unwanted side effects. It could make people's mouths and eyes become dry, and could cause constipation and blurred vision. It also sometimes made them drowsy, dizzy, and anxious, or gave them headaches. While these side effects were certainly less severe than those caused by iproniazid, many doctors weren't satisfied and continued their search for a better drug to treat depression.

In the 1980s, the SSRIs were created. Although they proved highly effective in many cases, they too had side effects. Prozac, for example, was the first major SSRI, appearing on the market in late 1987. It was such a success that within three years, its annual sales neared $800 million. However, the *Physician's Desk Reference* (PDR) says that Prozac's side effects may include abnormal dreams, abnormal ejaculation, abnormal vision, anxiety, diarrhea, diminished sex drive, dizziness, dry mouth, flu-like symptoms, flushing, gas, headache, impotence, insomnia, itching, loss of appetite, nausea, nervousness, rash, sex-drive changes, sinusitis, sleepiness, sore

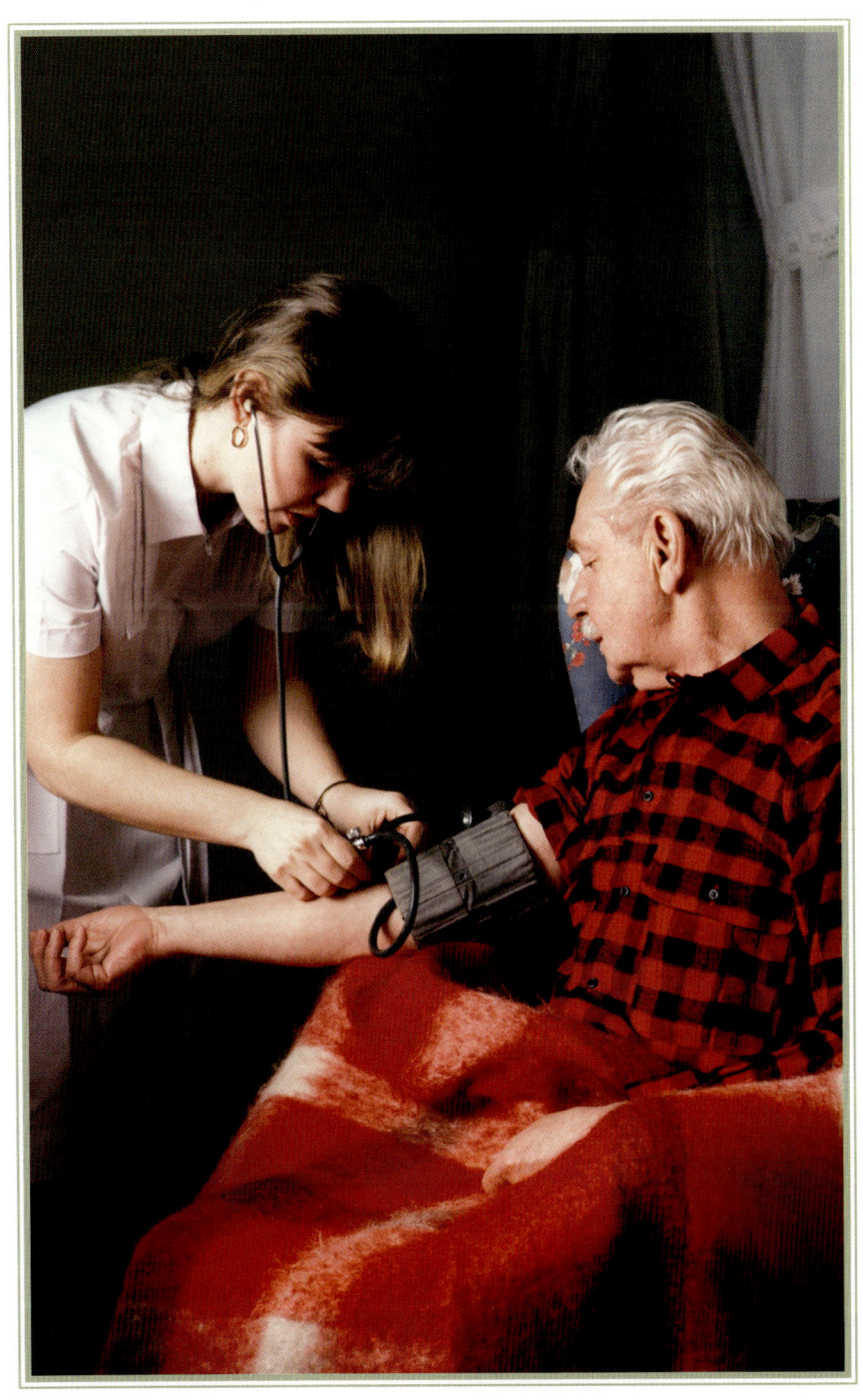

Iproniazid caused high blood pressure.

throat, sweating, tremors, upset stomach, vomiting, weakness, and yawning. The PDR also specifically points out that "side effects cannot be anticipated." This inability of anyone to predict or anticipate side effects is true of all SSRI antidepressants.

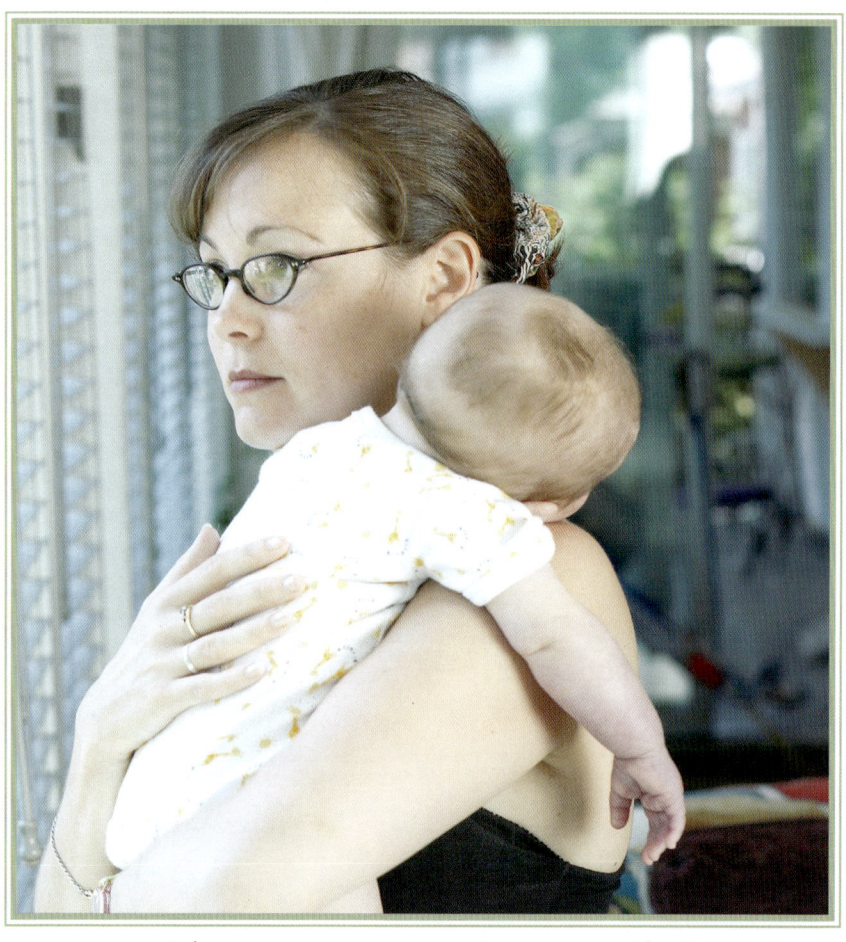

Antidepressants are sometimes prescribed to a woman experiencing postpartum depression. Because a mother needs to be able to adequately care for her baby, treating her depression is vital.

Some people, like Brooke Shields, find that the side effects they experience while taking an antidepressant are relatively mild. For example, one patient said, "I cleaned my house for days when I first went on Zoloft." Others may experience few if any side effects, while still others may simply find antidepressants uncomfortable and not very helpful. Zachary Howard took Zoloft for just one month in high school before stopping. "All it did was make me feel like I had no emotions. I felt like a zombie."

Others, however, have stronger reactions. Rebekah Beddoe started taking Zoloft shortly after giving birth to her first child. Her doctor suspected she suffered from postpartum depression and gave her a trial package of the antidepressant. "His words to me were, 'They're completely safe, very effective and only work on people with depression.' If he were to take them, he said, they'd do nothing because they just correct chemical imbalance."

At first Rebekah didn't want to be on drugs and didn't take them, but after a second doctor diagnosed her with depression, she changed her mind. A week later, however, while waiting for her group therapy session to begin, she suddenly found herself unable to breathe. She felt like the walls were closing in on her, and her heart was pounding so hard she was afraid she was having a heart attack. It was, instead, an *anxiety attack*—an extremely rare side effect of some antidepressants.

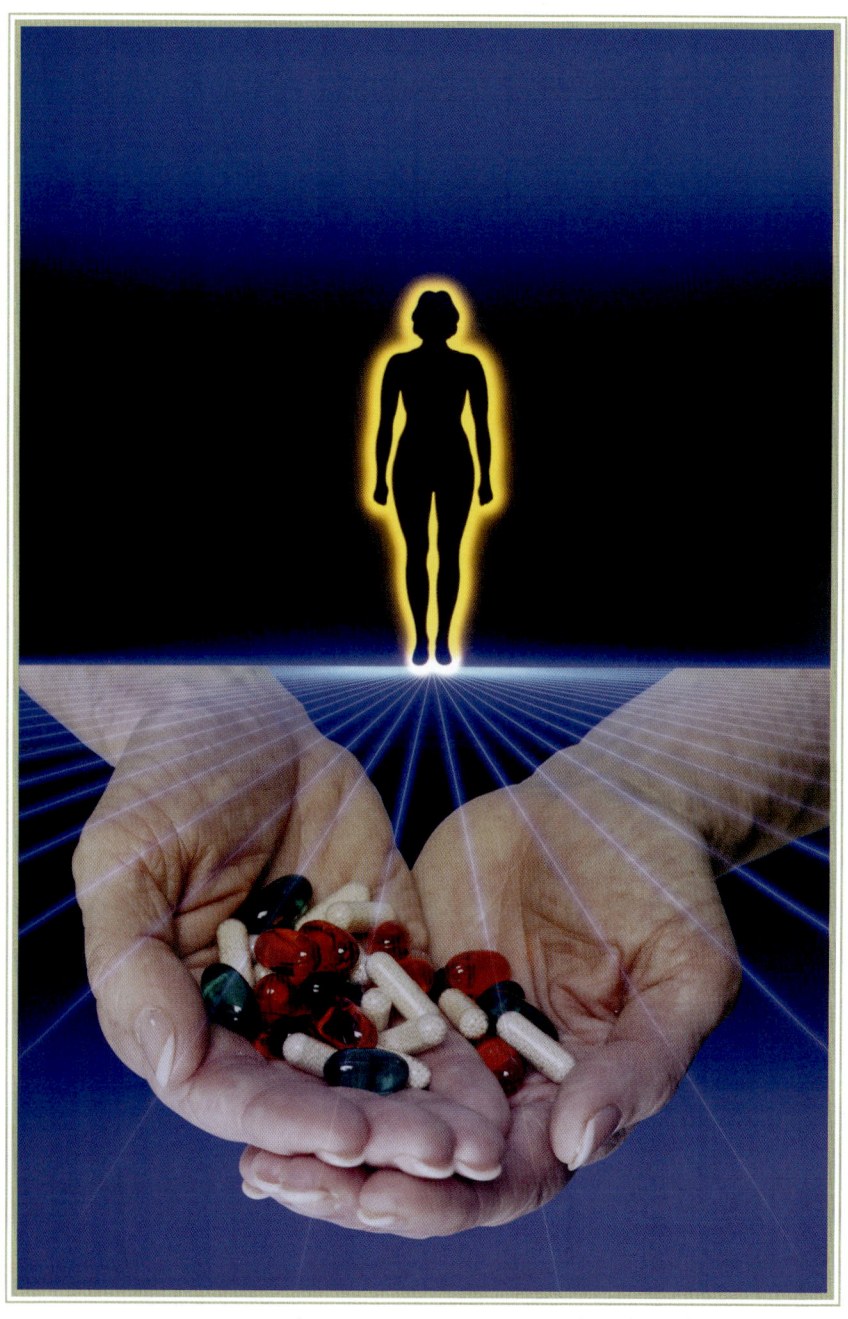

Despite antidepressants' potential side effects, some physicians and their patients consider antidepressants true miracle drugs.

The Benefits of Antidepressants

Antidepressants can be very effective in helping people cope with depression. John Lochridge, a child and adolescent psychiatrist in Smyrna, Georgia, calls Prozac "one of the top ten inventions of the twentieth century.... When it's prescribed right, it's a miracle. I've got 200 kids on an antidepressant right now, and if people took them away, I'd have parents up in arms, rioting in the streets." And Irl Extein, who has been practicing psychiatry for twenty years, adds, "In many cases they're miraculous and lifesaving." At the same time, however, it's possible that along with those benefits come uncomfortable side effects, forcing patients to ask themselves if the benefits of the drug are worth the possible side effects—and the potential risks.

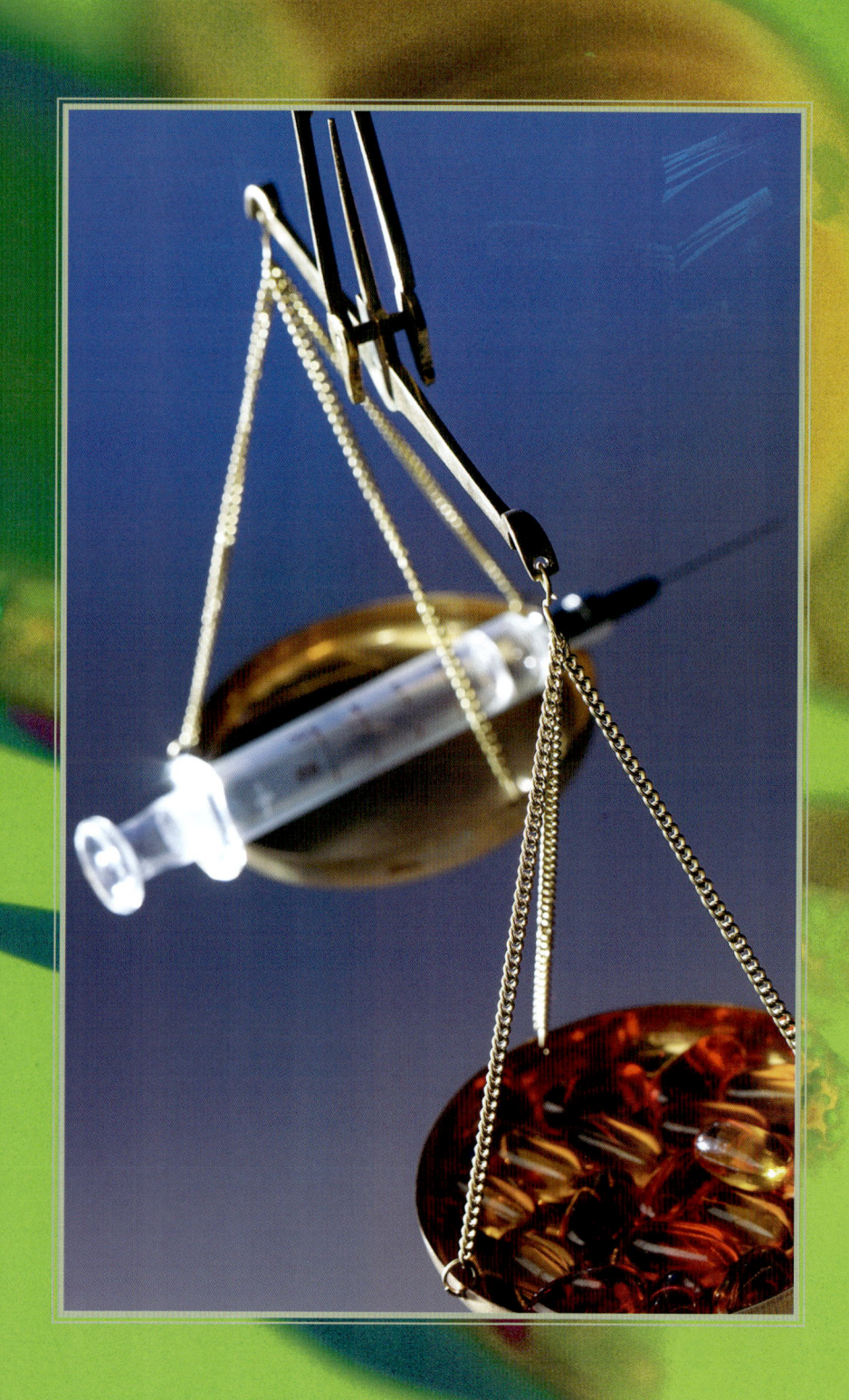

Chapter 2

Weighing Risks and Benefits

Thirteen-year-old Matthew Miller was very unhappy. Nine months earlier, his family had moved to a new neighborhood, and he had begun attending a new school. Under these circumstances, it's perhaps not surprising that he had become moody and withdrawn. It worried his teachers, however. His grades were lower than the teachers thought they should be, and the teachers were concerned that his withdrawal was more than just a passing teenage phase. They suggested his parents talk to a psychiatrist.

Matthew's parents took his teachers' advice. The psychiatrist ruled out ***attention deficit disorder***, but he made no

26   Antidepressants and Their Side Effects

other diagnosis. He did, however, give Matthew a three-week supply of Zoloft. He told Matthew's parents to have their son try the pills for a week, and then to get back to him.

The day before they were to see the psychiatrist again, Matthew seemed very **hyperactive**. According to his father, writing on the Web site www.drugawareness.org/Archives/Survivors/record0216.html, "his sister complained that Matt was being loud and bothering her more than normal. His grand-

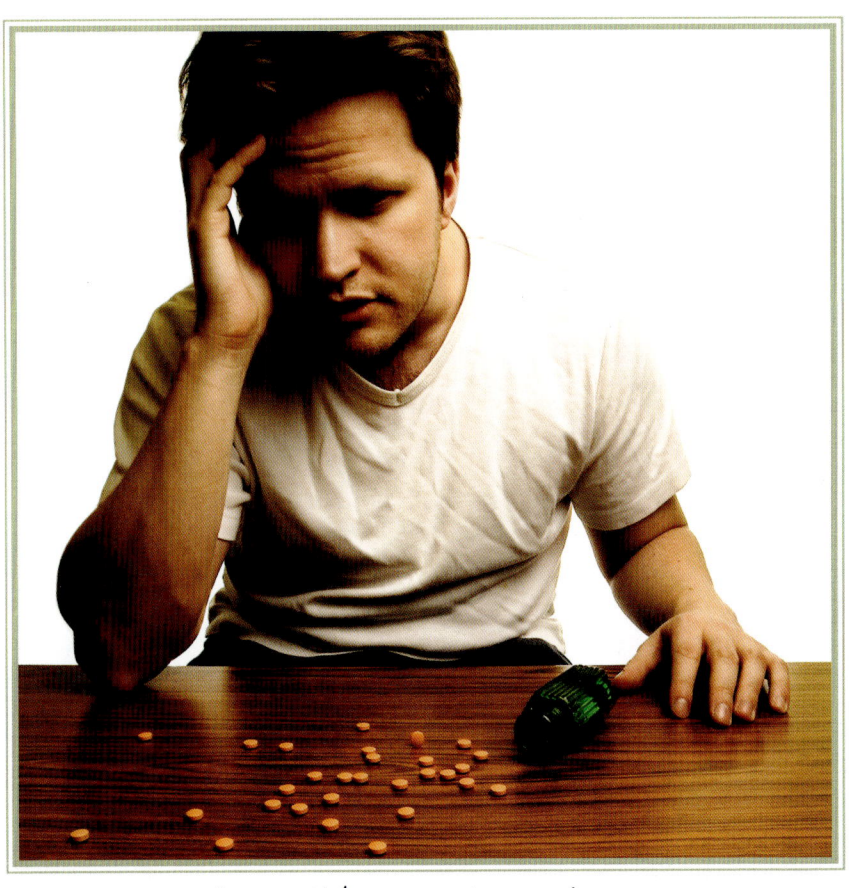

Using antidepressants may increase the likelihood of suicide.

mother . . . remarked that Matt could hardly sit still through our Sunday brunch."

That night, he hanged himself in his bedroom closet.

Antidepressants and Suicide

What happened to Matthew is an extreme example of the risks of antidepressants. Nonetheless, an increased tendency to commit suicide is one of the possibilities people taking antidepressants should consider. An analysis of twenty-five studies involving 4,600 children and teenagers showed that taking antidepressants doubled the risk of suicidal thoughts. As a result, the Food and Drug Administration (FDA) announced in the summer of 2004 that, because of this increased risk of suicidal thoughts, the packaging of all SSRIs should carry a "black box" warning, which is their strongest caution for prescription drugs. "Half of all kids who suffer from depression will attempt suicide at least once, and at least seven percent will die as a result," said Dr. David Fassler, a trustee of the American Psychiatric Association. "Every suicide is a tragedy, and any increased risk of suicidal thoughts or behaviors—no matter how small—must be taken seriously."

Coping with Side Effects

While most side effects of antidepressants are relatively minor, they can have a major effect on the lives of those taking them. People then have to decide if the benefits they receive are worth the drawbacks. Mimi Harrison, for instance, a writer in Washington D.C., quit Prozac because of its side effects. It made her "so agitated I felt like ants were crawling under my skin—and it did nothing for my symptoms."

Harrison switched from Prozac to Paxil, another of the major SSRIs. "After several weeks the drug kicked in," she wrote, "and, for the first time in memory, I could wake in the morning and open my eyes right away. . . . I no longer had to check my watch compulsively to account for every minute of my time. After a month of taking Paxil, I could mail letters easily and not obsess that they were deals with the devil; read the newspaper and not fear I had somehow caused the bedlam in the headlines; pass strangers on the street and not worry I

The Food and Drug Administration

The Food and Drug Administration (FDA) began with a single chemist employed by the Department of Agriculture in 1862. By 2001, it had more than 9,100 employees and a budget of almost $1.3 billion. The FDA oversees the manufacture, import, transport, storage, and sale of about $1 trillion worth of products every year. At first, the Division of Chemistry, as it was originally known, was purely scientific. Early in the twentieth century, however, that changed upon the publication of Upton Sinclair's novel The Jungle, *which detailed the nauseating conditions of the meatpacking industry. The public outcry was so great that a law was passed to guarantee the purity of the country's food, and the FDA was charged with this task. By the 1930s, the FDA began focusing on the country's increasing supply of drugs as well.*

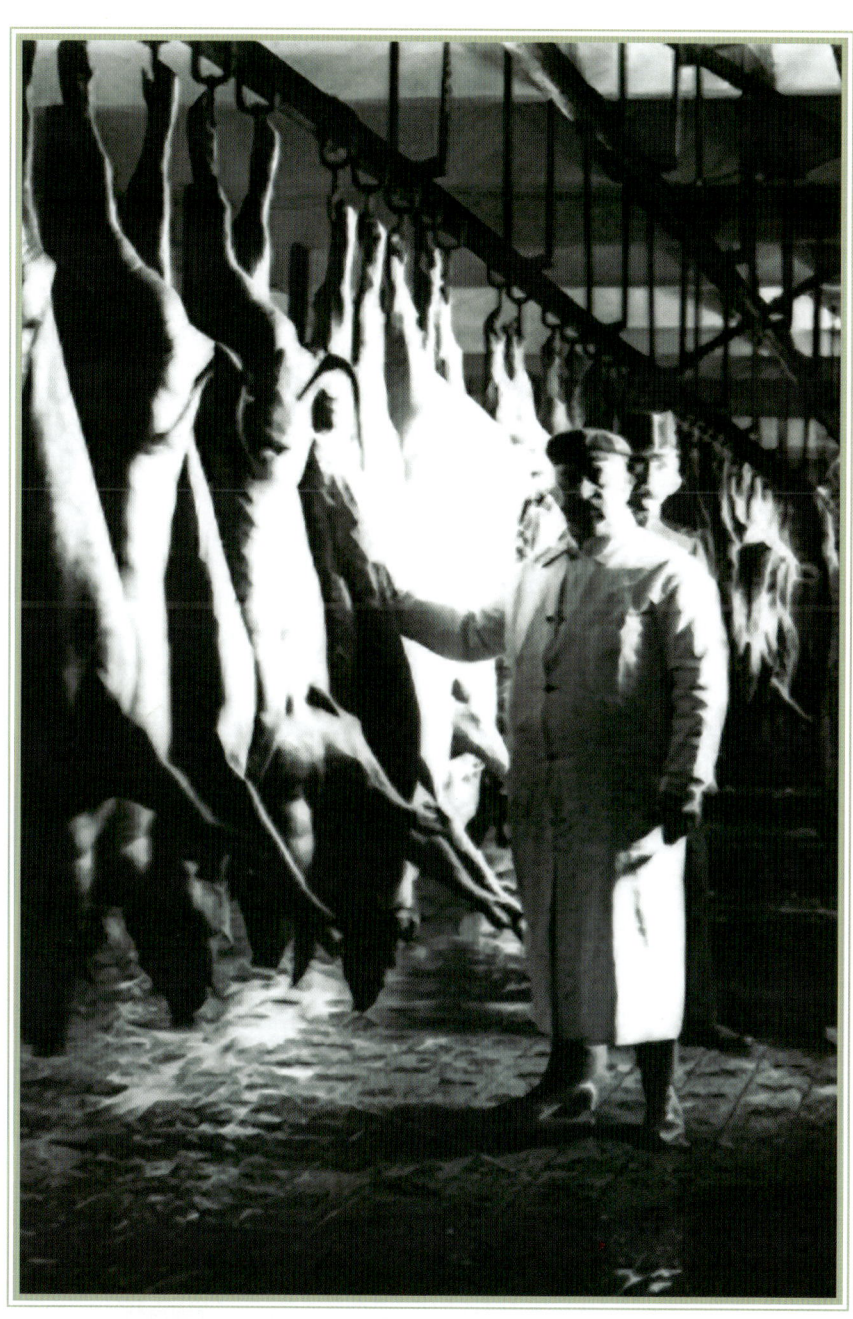

Upton Sinclair publicized the meatpacking industry's horrible conditions, which contributed to the development of the FDA.

had committed crimes against them or conspired to commit crimes with them. And, amazingly, I felt no side effects."

That didn't mean, however, that there weren't any. "It took me about six months," she wrote, "to notice I was eating a lot of sweets." Slowly but surely, she went from wearing a size 8 dress to a size 12. She told her doctor about her weight gain, but neither he nor she seemed too worried about it. "After all," she wrote, "what were a few extra pounds on my skinny body compared with the new life Paxil had given me?"

In 2000, after she had taken the drug for almost seven years, she noticed a new side effect. She had developed tremors in her hands, and now and then her arms and legs would jerk involuntarily. This extremely rare side effect didn't matter to her either. "Living with tremors," she wrote, "like being overweight, was a fair trade-off for the silence in my mind."

Unfortunately, she kept eating too much. According to Michael Jenike, a professor at Harvard, SSRIs are "more likely to cause weight gain than any other class of antidepressants," and "Paxil is by far the worst." (Other experts, however, disagree and point to tricyclics as being much worse than any SSRI.) Harrison wrote that while she did eat healthy things like fruits and nuts, she ate them "by the bowlful, and slice after slice of whole grain bread." She also ate cookies—lots of cookies. "Three were never enough," she wrote, "and ten were never too many. One night, as I stood in my kitchen staring down a bag of Milanos, I realized that it might as well have been a pack of cigarettes or a bottle of scotch." However, when she finally went to a gym to start working out, she was

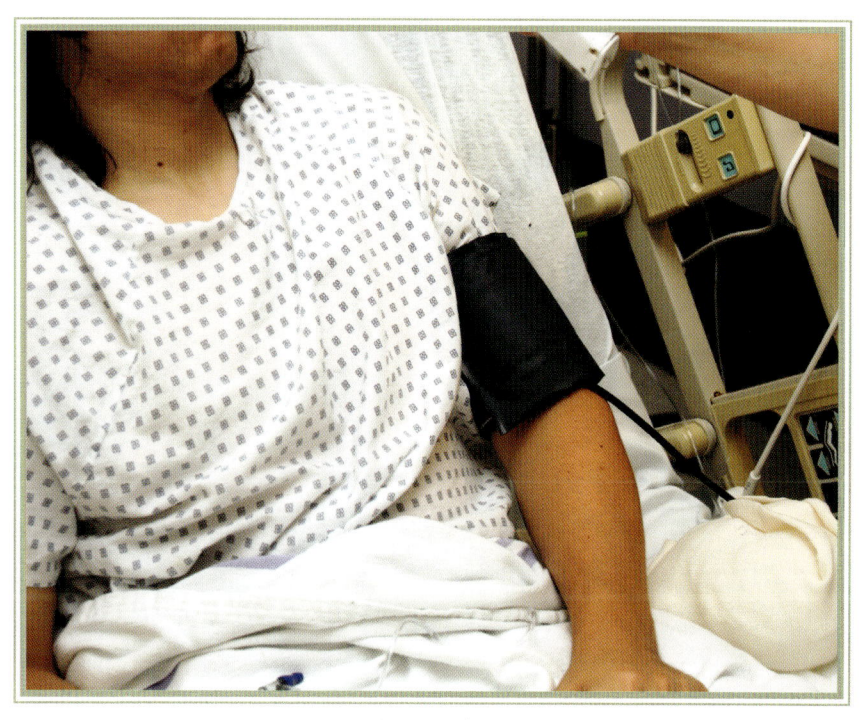

Long-term use of Paxil may have contributed to one individual's weight gain, which in turn led to her high blood pressure. She blamed the SSRI for her health issues.

turned away. Her blood pressure was higher than the gym's rules would allow. Also, she learned that her blood cholesterol count had climbed to a very high 268.

She finally managed to lose weight and to reduce both her blood pressure and cholesterol. But she wrote that she is "keenly aware that the normalcy I enjoy now may be borrowed. No one knows if long-term use of Paxil will damage my body, and I worry that the drug's beneficial effect on my brain chemistry will diminish over time."

Cholesterol

Cholesterol is a fatty steroid found in the bodies of animals. Because it does not dissolve in water, it builds up in the blood vessels of people who eat animal products like meat and milk. Sometimes this buildup causes arteriosclerosis, or hardening of the arteries, which makes it more difficult for the heart to pump blood through the body. If the arteries around the heart harden, this can cause heart disease. If the arteries in the leg harden, a person may have difficulty walking. An excess of cholesterol might also cause a clot to form in the blood. If this clot breaks loose and travels into the heart, it will cause a heart attack. It if travels into the brain, it causes a stroke.

When Coping Is Impossible

The side effects Angela Bolin claimed she experienced from taking Paxil were much more severe. She started taking the medication in the summer of 2002, and she was sure she began noticing side effects just a few days later. For example, she found herself disagreeing with people frequently. She would cry for no reason and even claw at herself. Once, when she was having an argument with her parents, she started banging her head against the wall so much that her father had to stop her. She says that when she told her psychiatrist about the incident, the doctor suggested doubling the dosage of the drug. Once she walked into a store at the mall and bought

Weighing Risks and Benefits 33

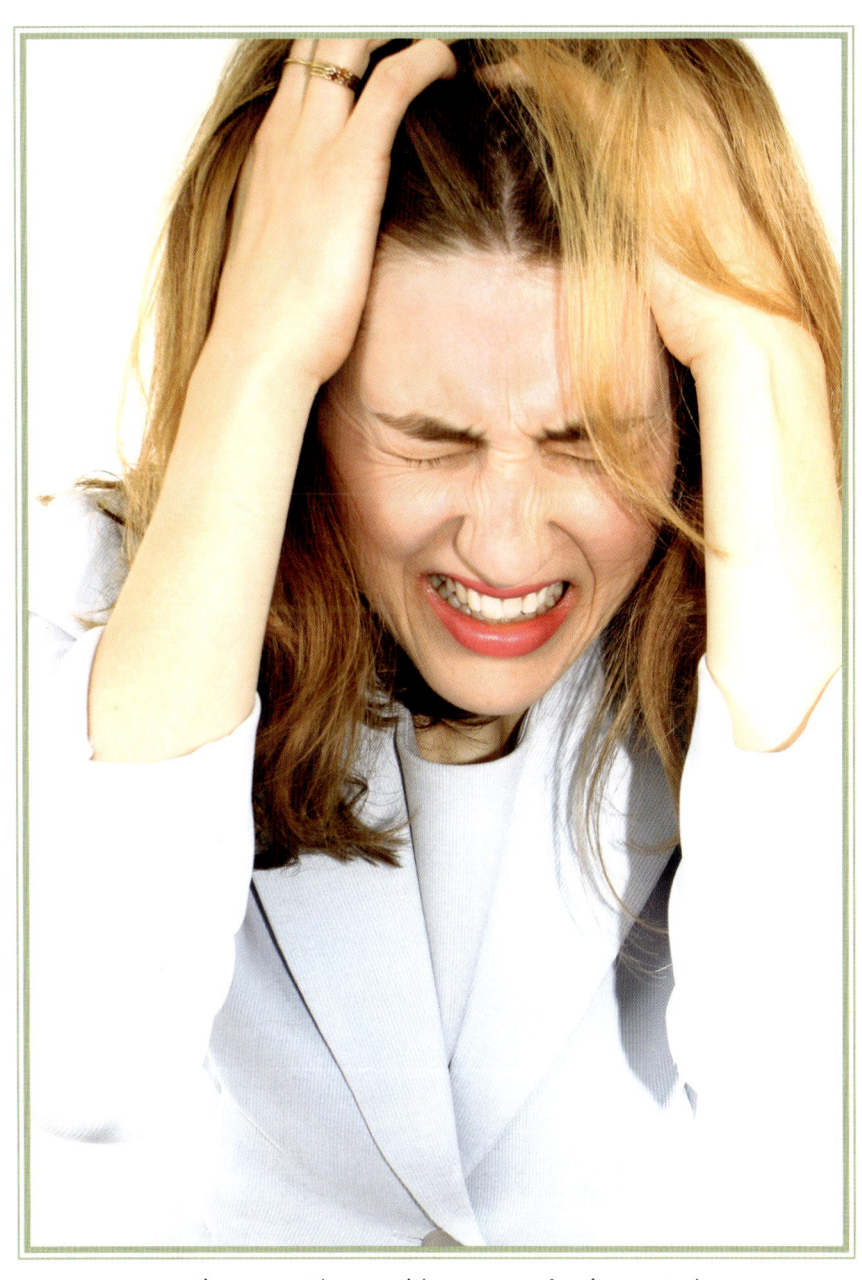

Another Paxil user blames it for her violent emotions. This is a case where the question must be asked: which came first, the chicken or the egg (her emotions or the medication)?

34   Antidepressants and Their Side Effects

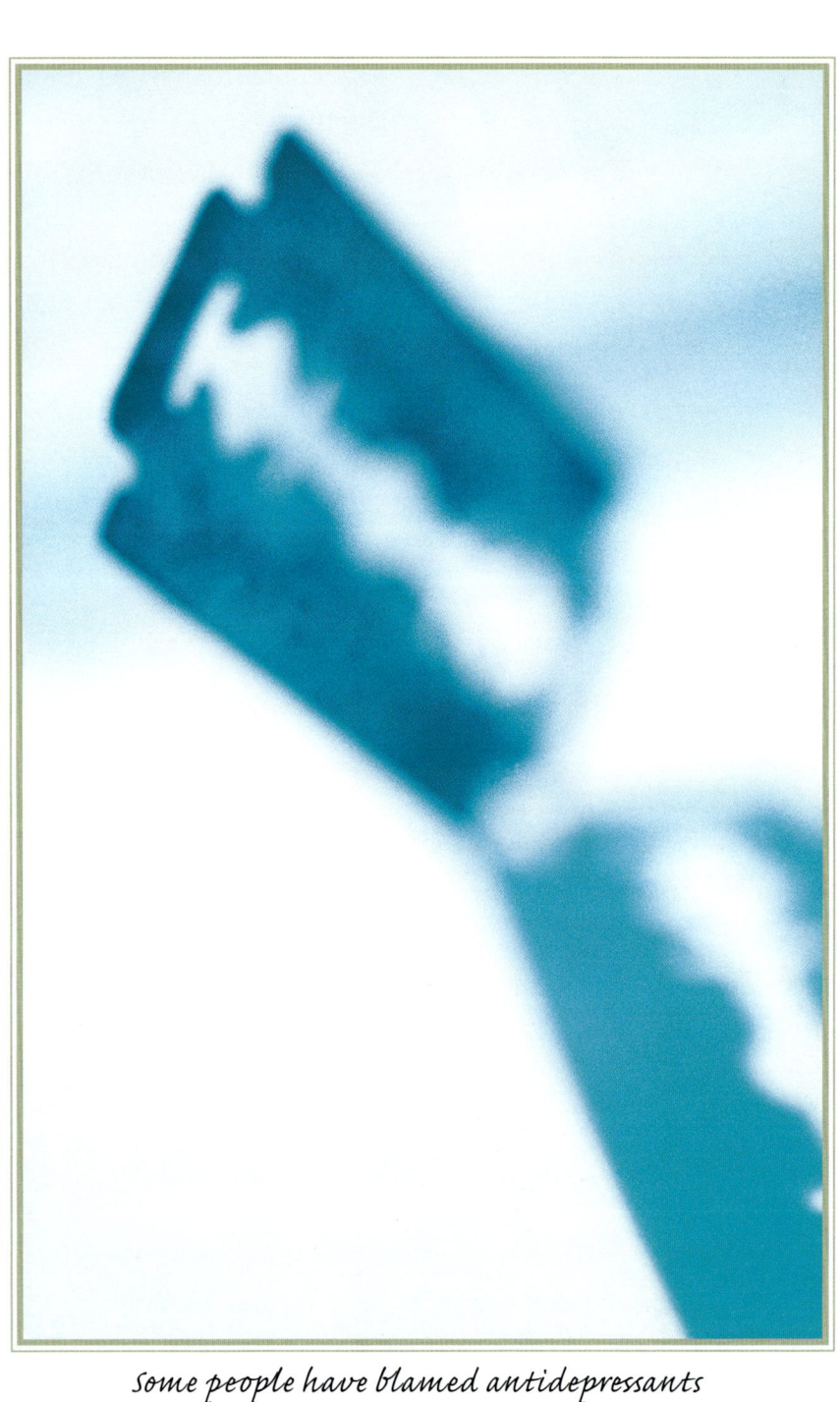

Some people have blamed antidepressants for making them suicidal.

nearly every product in the store. Another time, she stood in a bed of fire ants without moving. And one day, she left campus early so that she could buy razors to cut herself with.

That night at dinner, her father told her she shouldn't be on Paxil. That made her angry, so she went upstairs into her room and started systematically cutting herself with those razors: cut to the left leg, and then one on the right leg, moving toward her knees. She later said she felt as though she was watching a movie and had no control over her actions. Finally, she passed out from loss of blood.

She tried to kill herself again, cutting herself more than 200 times in the bathroom of a department store. She ended up being hospitalized in two mental institutions and had to

Prescription Drug Use in the United States

In 2004, the Department of Health and Human Services reported that almost half of all Americans were taking at least one prescription drug, and that one in six was taking three or more. This represented a 13 percent increase over the number who were taking at least one drug in 1994 and a 40 percent increase in those taking three or more. Five out of every six people over the age of sixty-five took at least one prescription drug every day. Almost half took three or more. Adult use of antidepressants almost tripled between 1994 and 2000. Ten percent of women and 4 percent of men over the age of eighteen take them.

drop out of college. Luckily, she managed to recover. She and her fiancé moved to Florida in 2003, and she no longer takes antidepressants. For her, the benefits were simply not worth it. "I can never be the person I was before," she said. "But I want to try to get back to where I was."

Although Angela Bolin blames Paxil for her problems, most psychiatrists don't take her claim very seriously. Instead, they believe it was mere coincidence that Bolin was on Paxil at the same time that she was experiencing severe psychiatric symptoms. These symptoms are typical of a personality disorder; in all likelihood, Paxil did not cause her behaviors or even make them worse.

Camille Stallings started taking Paxil when she was sixteen years old. Not only did her depression remain, she also gained thirty pounds. When she tried to stop taking the drug, she would become dizzy and almost pass out. She changed to another antidepressant called Wellbutrin® (bupropion), but the only thing that changed was her weight. She began purging after her meals and dropped to ninety-five pounds. Then she tried a third antidepressant. This one was called Celexa, but that only made her feel numb.

Camille finally decided that antidepressants weren't for her. In an article in the *Washington Times*, she is quoted: "What the doctor put me through was just ridiculous, And I don't think that's unusual. Pretty much all you have to do is say, 'I struggle with anxiety,' and they'll prescribe you something."

In 2005, Camille turned twenty-five years old. A counselor began to help her deal with her depression, but she had lost

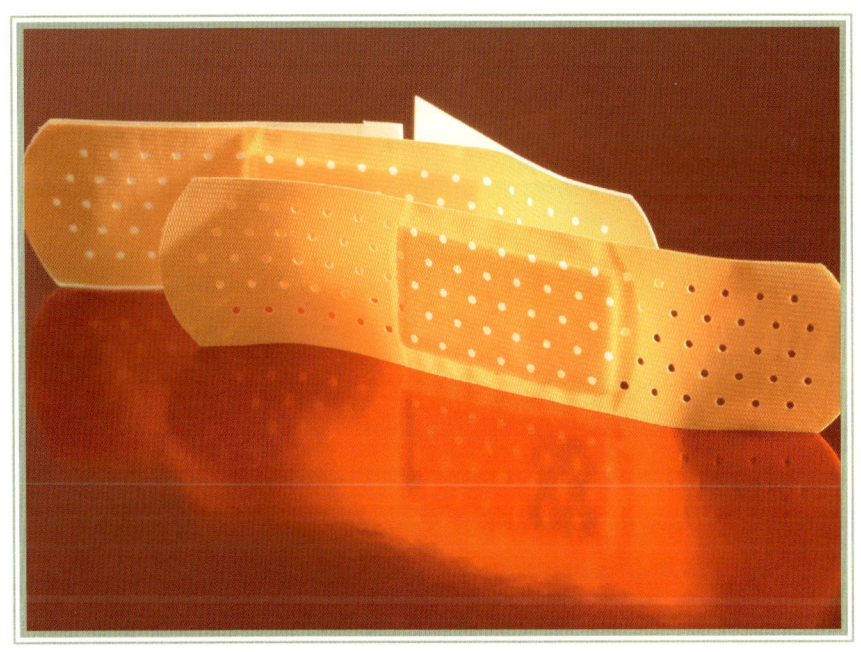

If a person tries to take antidepressants as a way to avoid painful personal issues, it may be like slapping a Band-Aid over a deep wound.

faith in antidepressants. "They never took care of the root problem of my depression," she said. "It's like putting a Band-Aid over a huge cut."

Different Viewpoints

Of course, not everyone agrees with her. Chris Duplisea, a twenty-three-year-old elementary school teacher, said that he found antidepressants "liberating." After he moved twelve times in one year and broke up with his girlfriend, he became so anxious and depressed that he couldn't give spelling tests in class or even make photocopies of his class assignments. He also found it difficult to eat.

"You just want to tear yourself out of your skin," he said in a *Washington Times* article. "You just want to run and scream."

Finally he decided to see a psychiatrist. He was a little worried at first. "I didn't know if I'd walk in there and see people drooling, whacking their heads off the wall," he said. "You think of psychiatrists, and you think of wackos . . . a mental ward. [But] when I got in there, and it was a bunch of normal people in there, it was OK."

His doctor prescribed Lexapro® (escitalopram) for him, and it made a difference in his life right away. "A lot of what these medicines do is they just put your feet on the ground," he said. "It clears your mind enough so you can start thinking normally again to fix the problem."

Sexual Side Effects

Perhaps one of the more troublesome aspects of antidepressants is the risk of sexual side effects. These occur in 60 percent of men and women who take them. Some of these side effects include decreased sexual desire (libido), impotence, delayed ejaculation, and diminished ability to have an orgasm.

Sharon, for instance, was a woman much like many others. In her mid-thirties, she was married with two children and also had a career as a freelance journalist. Depression, however, was beginning to interfere with her work. It was also making her very irritable and distancing her from her

Weighing Risks and Benefits 39

two daughters. Worried, she started taking 20 milligrams of Prozac every day.

It did improve her mood, her energy, and her concentration. At the same time, however, she began encountering a problem she had never had before. "In the two months I've been on Prozac," she told her psychiatrist, "having an orgasm just became more and more difficult, until now it's impossible. Climaxing took more intense stimulation for longer and longer periods of time: five minutes became ten minutes,

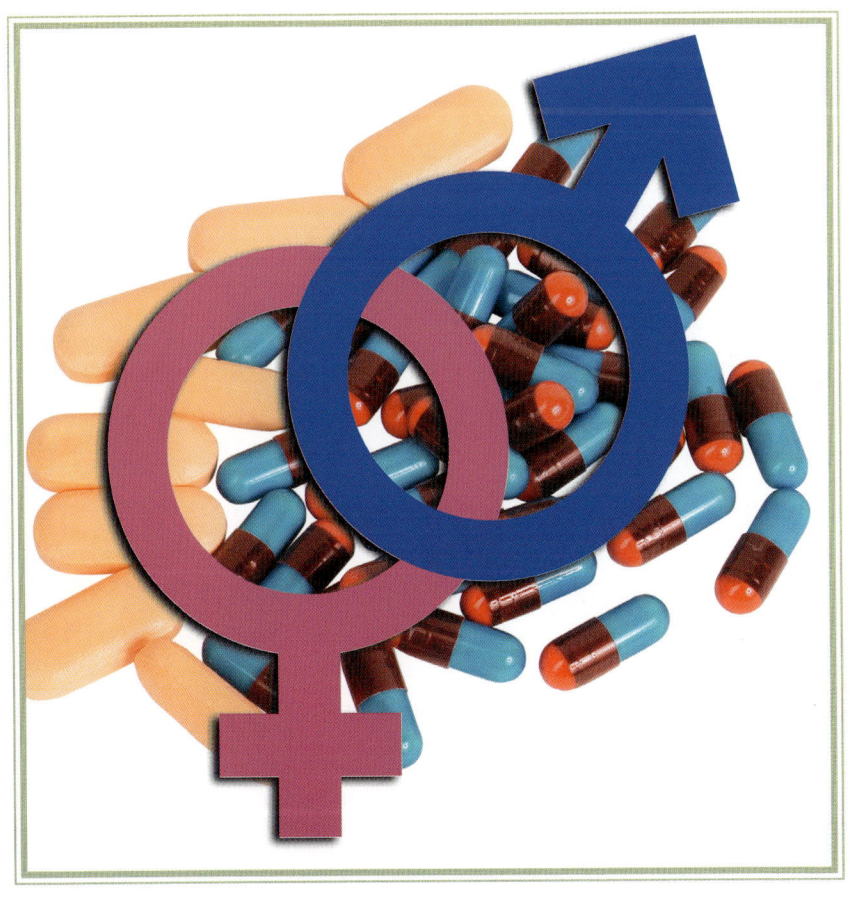

Antidepressants can affect sexual desire.

became thirty minutes, and eventually I couldn't at all." And what made it even more frustrating was that, since the drug relieved her depression, she was more interested in sex than she had been before.

At first, she thought the relief from depression was worth putting up with these side effects. When asked if she wanted to stay on antidepressants, she replied, "Yes. I've still got four major articles due in the next six months. I can't afford to get depressed again. The kids are so much happier with me feeling better. I can't go off the medication right now."

She and her doctor began searching for another antidepressant, one that would relieve her depression but not have

Wellbutrin

Wellburtrin (bupropion) is neither a tricyclic nor an SSRI. It has a different chemical structure than the tricyclics, and instead of suppressing the reabsorption of serotonin, as the SSRIs do, it suppresses the reabsorption of the neurotransmitters norepinephrine and dopamine. Like all antidepressants, it can cause unanticipated side effects. These include agitation, constipation, dizziness, dry mouth, excessive sweating, headache, nausea, vomiting, skin rash, sleep disturbances, and tremors. When Wellbutrin is being taken by somehow who is purging, there is considerable danger of seizures. However, Wellbutrin appears to cause fewer sexual side effects than SSRIs.

those sexual side effects. First she went to Zoloft and then to Serzone®, a non-SSRI, but she had essentially the same response. Finally she tried Wellbutrin, another non-SSRI. This finally gave her the combination of relief with no side effects that she'd been searching for.

No Magic Pill

Using antidepressants will not magically solve a person's every problem. However, a study released in early 2006 indicated that antidepressants brought complete relief to about 30 percent of the people who took them, 60 to 70 percent showed some improvement, and the rest were not helped significantly. Unfortunately, no one can predict for sure what side effects an antidepressant may have. They may be relatively minor, like nausea, or they may be major, like thoughts of suicide.

But perhaps the most frightening possible side effect is the chance that antidepressants may turn people into murderers.

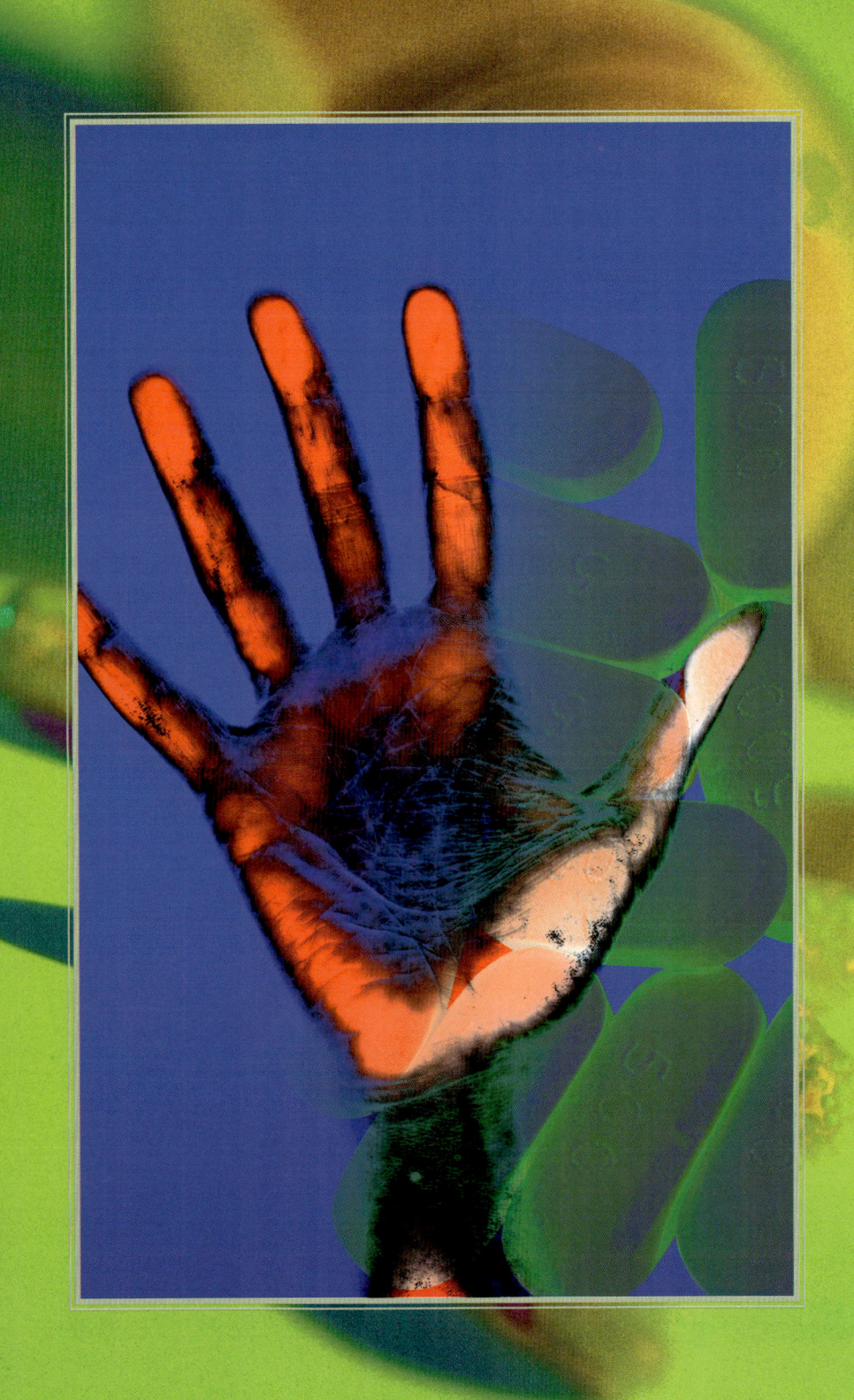

Chapter 3

Antidepressants and Violence: Fact or Excuse?

On April 20, 1999, Eric Harris and Dylan Klebold opened fire on their fellow students at Columbine High School in Littleton, Colorado, killing thirteen people and injuring twenty-four others before turning their guns on themselves and committing suicide. It was the worst school massacre in U.S. history.

Mark Taylor, nineteen years old at the time, was one of the victims:

> I was sitting on a hill outside the school eating lunch with my best friend "when Eric Harris came over and started shooting me. I was shot between seven and thirteen times. No one really knows the exact number because there were so many

43

bullet tracks. Most of the bullets just went right through me. After I was shot I just lay there, playing dead, and could see others being shot.

Mark spent two months in the hospital and over the next three years endured several operations as a result of the wounds he received that day.

But Mark did not blame Eric Harris for what he did. "Everybody thought Eric and Dylan were the nicest people," he said. "My cousin, who was in Eric's class, told me that Eric and Dylan used to bring her flowers and cookies. . . . I don't have ill feelings against him since I don't think you can hold him accountable." Instead, Mark blamed a company, Solvay Pharmaceuticals Inc., for what happened to him, and in 2003, he filed a lawsuit against them. "I'm suing Solvay," he said, "because I believe that Eric Harris did what he did because of this drug." Mark later dropped the lawsuit.

Antidepressants and Teen Violence

Solvay is the manufacturer of Luvox, the antidepressant that Harris was taking at the time of the shootings. The PDR says that about 4 percent of people who take Luvox develop manic reactions. (Mania is defined as "a form of psychosis characterized by exalted feelings, delusions of grandeur . . . and over-production of ideas.") According to court records in Colorado, Harris's prescription for Luvox had been filled ten times between April of 1998 and March of 1999. In December 1998, his dosage had been increased, and his autopsy revealed a "therapeutic level" of Luvox in his system when he died.

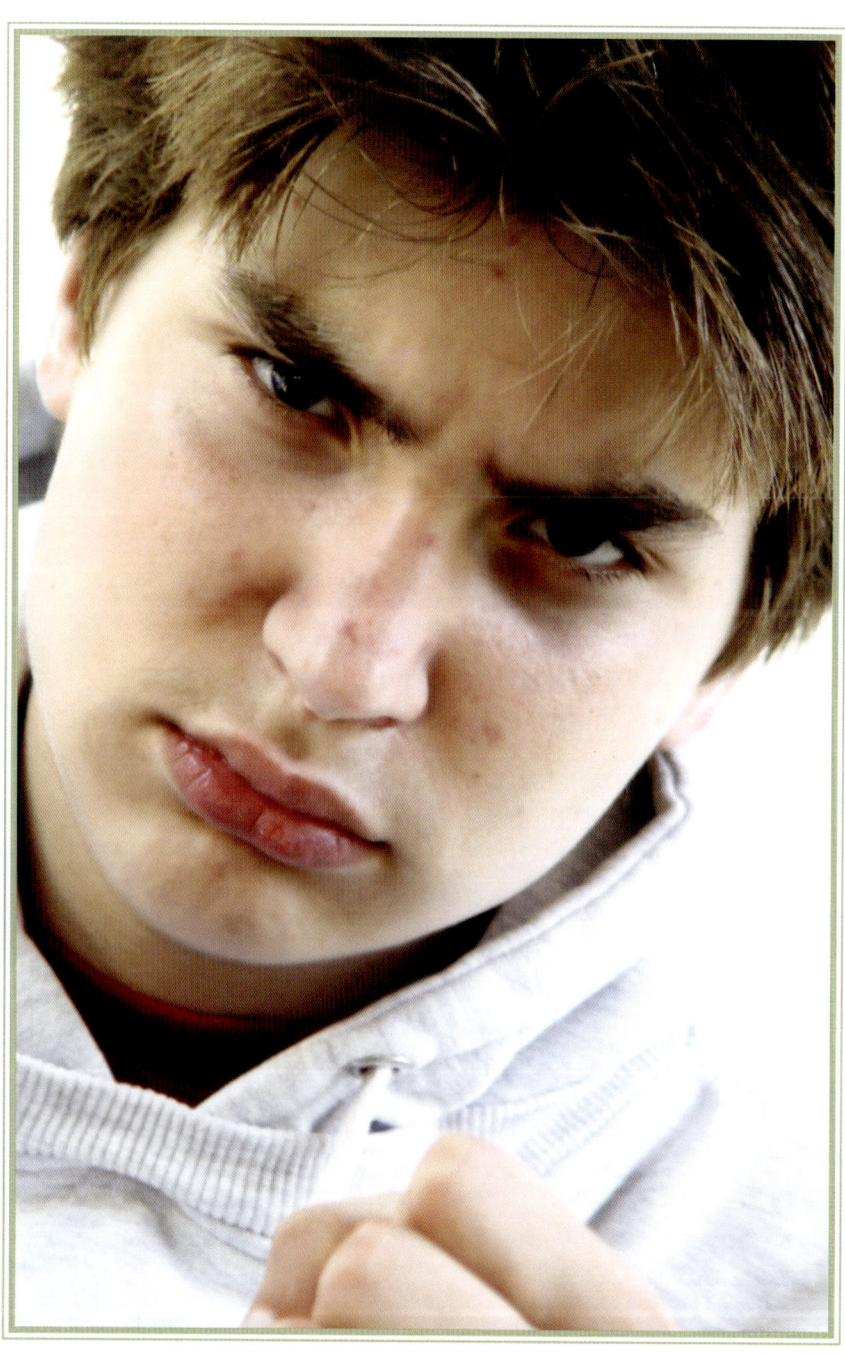

Rightly or wrongly, antidepressants have been blamed for incidents of teen violence.

Unfortunately, Eric Harris is not the only example of a young person on antidepressants becoming violent. In 1998, Kip Kinkel murdered his parents, then went to school and killed two more while wounding twenty-two. He was fifteen years old and was taking Prozac. In 2001, Jason Hoffman wounded a teacher and three students at his high school. Hoffman was eighteen and was taking two antidepressants: Effexor and Celexa. And in March 2005, sixteen-year-old Jeff Weise murdered his grandfather and his grandfather's companion before heading to school and killing ten more, including himself. Like Kinkel, he'd been taking Prozac. In fact, his aunts said that they had just recently upped his dosage from two pills a night to three.

After the Weise shooting, groups opposed to the use of antidepressants in children called on the FDA to investigate the relationship between antidepressants and these sorts of murders. Vera Hassner Sharav, the president of the Alliance for

Eli Lilly and Co.

Eli Lilly and Company was founded by Colonel Eli Lilly, a veteran of the Civil War, in May of 1876. Lilly was a thirty-eight-year-old pharmaceutical chemist who found the drugs of the time ineffective and poorly prepared. The company has grown from three employees in Indianapolis, Indiana, to 43,000 employees worldwide. More than 8,000 of these employees are engaged in the research and development of new drugs.

Human Research Protection, said that SSRIs interfere with a person's **inhibitions**.

"Lots of us have violent thoughts," she writes on the organization's Web site, "'I would like to take this man by the throat, he's bothering me.' But we don't do it. The drug removes that inhibition to act out and that is why you have these explosive situations."

However, John M. Plewes, medical adviser at Eli Lilly, the maker of Prozac, disagrees:

> That's just not a correct scientific statement. There is no credible scientific evidence that has established a causal connection between Prozac and either violent or suicidal behavior. This kind of behavior sometimes is a part of a serious, life-threatening illness—that illness can be depression or some other illnesses—but it's characterized by a variety of symptoms. And suicidal acts and thinking are symptoms of depression.

Certainly Jeff had had a difficult life. His father committed suicide in 1997, and two years later his mother was left brain-damaged by an automobile accident. A month before the shootings, he had tried to kill himself by slitting his wrists. But the question remains: would he have murdered these people if he hadn't been taking Prozac?

Antidepressants and Adult Violence

It's possible that antidepressants may inspire violence in adults, as well. In May of 1998, comedian and *Saturday Night*

Live veteran Phil Hartman was murdered in his sleep by his wife, Brynn. His wife, who committed suicide a few hours after killing her husband, was found to have alcohol, cocaine, and Zoloft in her body. According to Craig Harvey, the county coroner's investigator, "Between the cocaine and alcohol, the two of them most definitely intensified the other's effects. The Zoloft is kind of a wild card."

In the summer of 2001, Andrea Yates murdered her five children by drowning them in the bathtub. Two years earlier, she had become clinically depressed after the birth of her fourth child and tried to kill herself. She had been taking two antidepressants, Effexor and Remeron®, at the time of the murders.

Also in 2001, David John Hawkins strangled his wife of fifty years after taking 250 mg of Zoloft, five times the recom-

Coroner

A coroner is a public official, usually at the county or city level, whose job is to investigate any death that may not have been due to natural causes. The word "coroner" comes from the Middle English word for "officer of the crown." It dates from the twelfth century, when the coroner helped to investigate suspicious deaths. At one time, the coroner was responsible for all criminal proceedings. Today, many cities and counties in the United States have replaced the office of coroner with the office of medical examiner, who must also be a physician.

mended dose. The judge in the case, Barry O'Keefe, blamed the drug directly:

> The killing was totally out of character for the prisoner, inconsistent with the loving, caring relationship which existed between him and his wife and with their happy marriage of fifty years. I am satisfied that but for the Zoloft he had taken, he would not have strangled his wife.

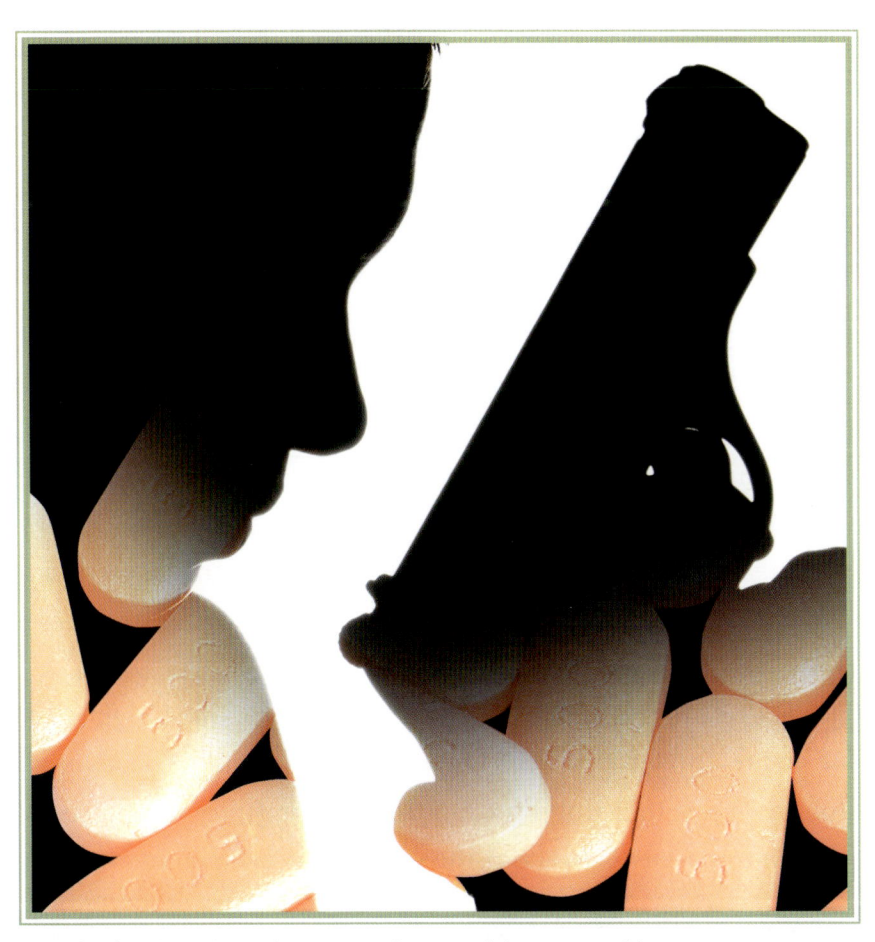

Both the legal and scientific worlds are still investigating the connection between violence and antidepressants.

An Adequate Excuse for Violence?

But not everyone is willing to put the blame on antidepressants. After all, the individuals in these stories were distressed and depressed prior to treatment with antidepressants. These were not ordinary people who suddenly turned into killers after taking an antidepressant; their behavior had been abnormal before treatment. In fact, their behaviors were one of the reasons why they were being treated in the first place.

In February 2005, a South Carolina jury found fifteen-year-old Christopher Pittman guilty of murdering his grandparents when he was twelve. Though he admitted he had killed them, his lawyers argued that because he was talking antidepressants, he didn't know what he was doing.

A month before the killings, Christopher was put on Paxil after he threatened to kill himself. After he moved in with his grandparents, another doctor put him on Zoloft. "We do not convict children for murder when they have been ambushed by chemicals that destroy their ability to reason," said his lawyer at the trial.

The final witness for the defense was Richard Kapit, who once handled applications and safety reviews of antidepressants at the FDA. He testified that Christopher's "whole sequence of actions was rash and frantic and done at a high level of anger—anger that was chemically induced." His lawyers told the jury that finding Christopher not guilty would send the nation a message about the dangers of antidepressants.

But the jury found him guilty, believing that he knew exactly what he was doing when he shot his grandparents, burned down their house, and then drove away in their car.

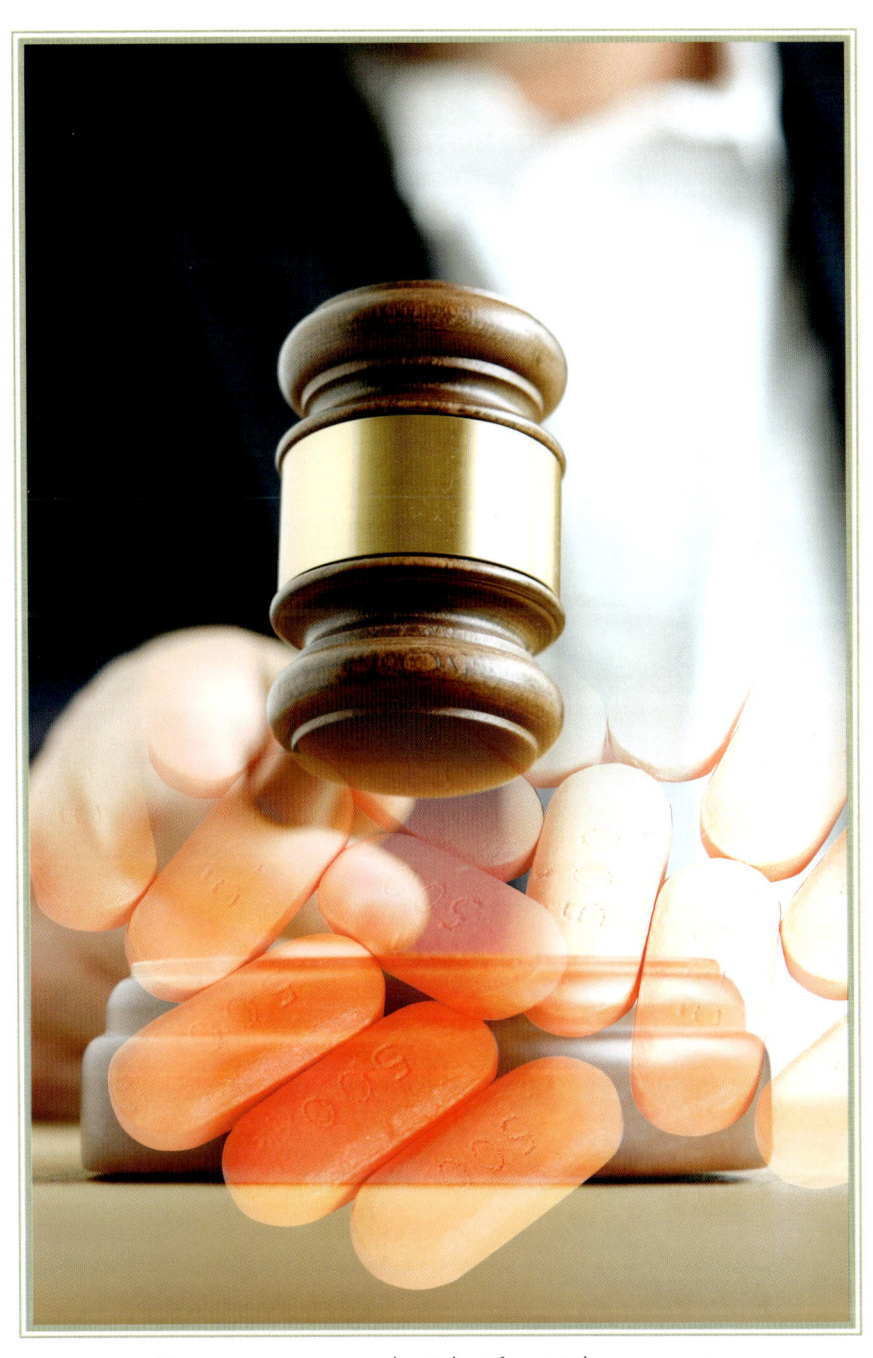

Antidepressants and Violence: Fact or Excuse? 51

The courts must decide if antidepressants offer a legal excuse for violence.

The judge in this case sentenced Christopher to fifteen to thirty years in prison.

Some people also claim that antidepressants are being used by the military to encourage them to kill. In early 2005, Jimmy Massey, a Marine from Waynesville, North Carolina, was interviewed by Patrizio Lombroso of the Italian newspaper *Il Manifesto*. Massey had served twelve years in the military and was a sergeant with the Third Marine Battalion when the United States invaded Iraq in the spring of 2003. After months of killing, however, he couldn't take it anymore. "I physically lost control of my **equilibrium** and couldn't move or talk," he said. "I stayed in one place and looked all the time at the wall. I was really scared, and lost."

He was diagnosed with major depressive disorder. "For three weeks in Iraq," he said, "they filled me with anti-depressives and psychotropic drugs. That's the emergency treatment

Psychotropic Drugs

All antidepressants are also psychotropic. A psychotropic drug is one that alters the perception, emotion, or behavior of the user. The antipsychotic drug Thorazine® (chlorpromazine), for example, is psychotropic. It is often used to treat people with schizophrenia. Other anti-psychotic drugs include Haldol® (haloperidol) and Clozaril® (clozapine). Psychotropic drugs like lithium can help people with bipolar disorder, while Librium® (chlordiazepoxide) can be useful in treating anxiety.

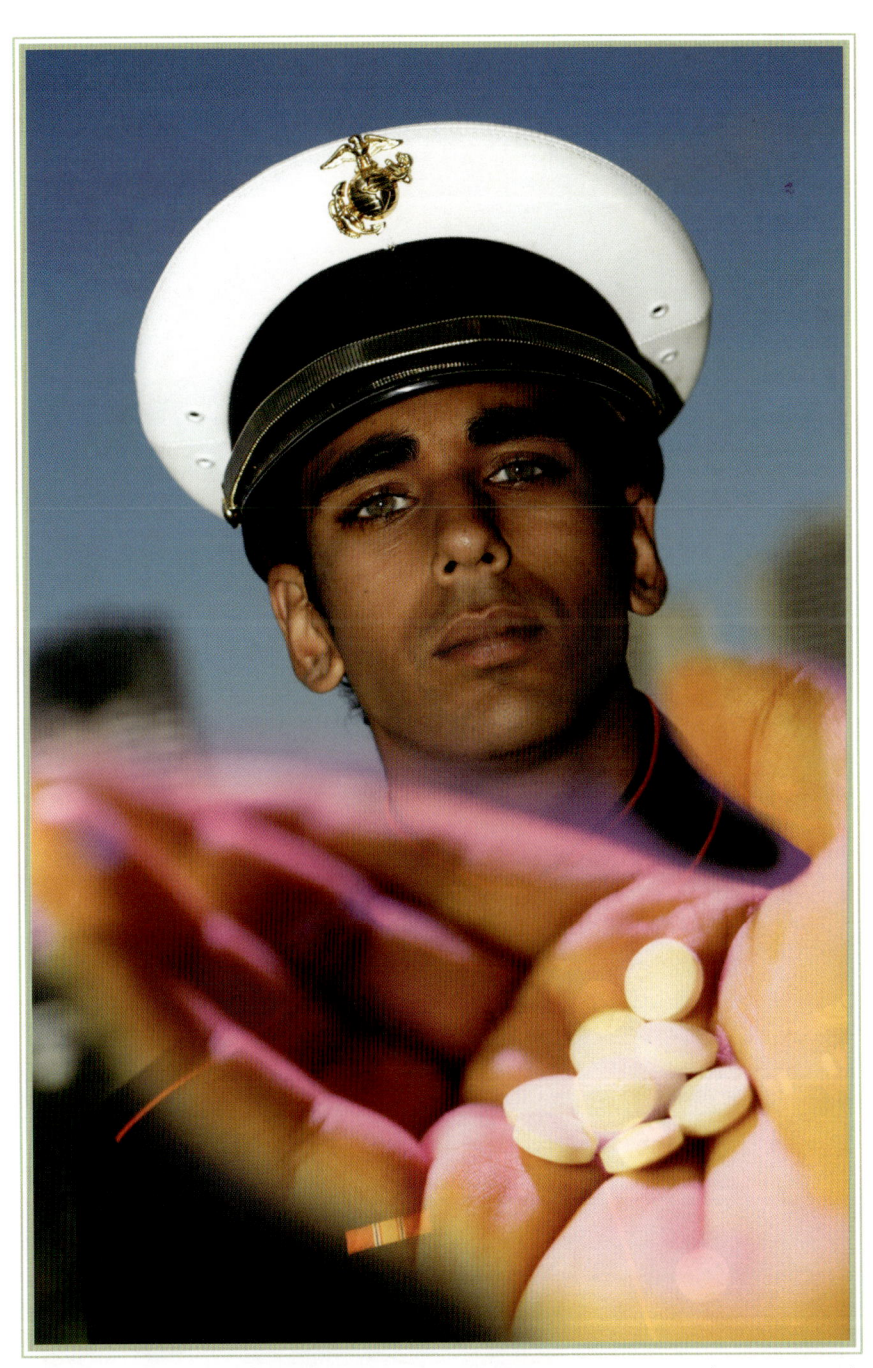

Antidepressants and Violence: Fact or Excuse?   53

Claims have been made that antidepressants are being used in the military to break down people's resistance to killing.

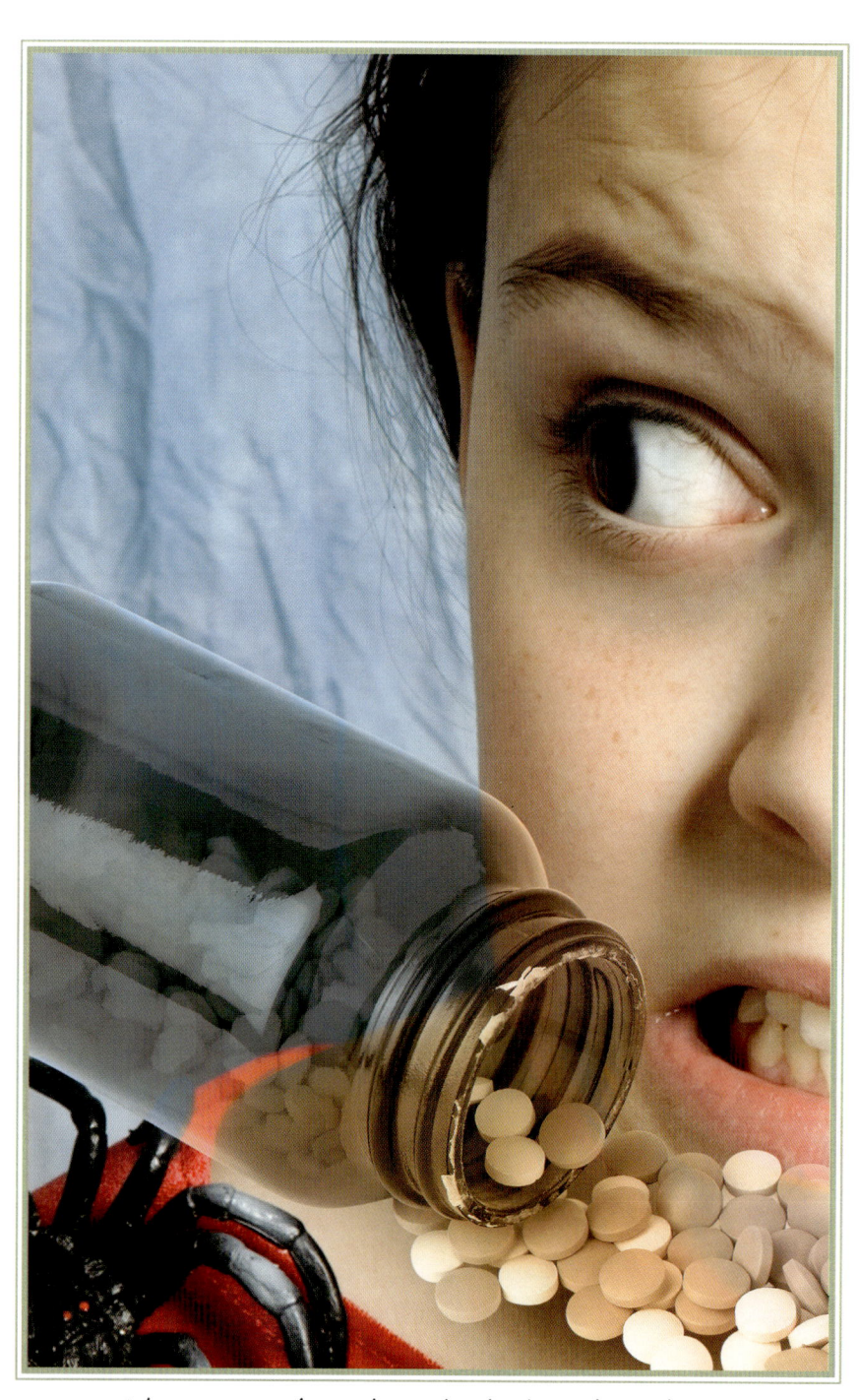

Antidepressants have been linked with nightmares.

for these cases of 'traumatic stress,' when the idea of refusing to kill takes over a soldier's life." But it didn't work for him. After three weeks, "they didn't know what to do and sent me back. Now I am out of the military, incapacitated and disabled, with an honorable discharge."

When Lombroso asked him if there were other Marines in the same situation, Massey said, "Many. And they are still at the front. They stuff them with anti-depressants, and after that they go back and are sent into combat again." He added that "in 2004, thirty-one Marines took their own lives, and eighty-five made suicide attempts. Most of those who wanted to die rather than keep on killing are less than twenty-five years old, and sixteen percent of them are under twenty years."

Self-Destruction—or Salvation?

Antidepressants may cause not just violence to others but also violence toward the self. A 2004 article in the Syracuse, New York, *Post Standard* relates two such instances.

One night, noises woke Valerie Kotyra from her sleep, and when she went downstairs to investigate, she found her twenty-four-year-old daughter, Rebecca Caraway, curled up on the floor in front of the refrigerator. Her face was red and her fists were clenched.

"Mommy, the spiders are coming," she said.

"Did you have a bad dream?" said her mother. "Did you see a spider?"

"No, I hear them coming. They're coming, Mommy."

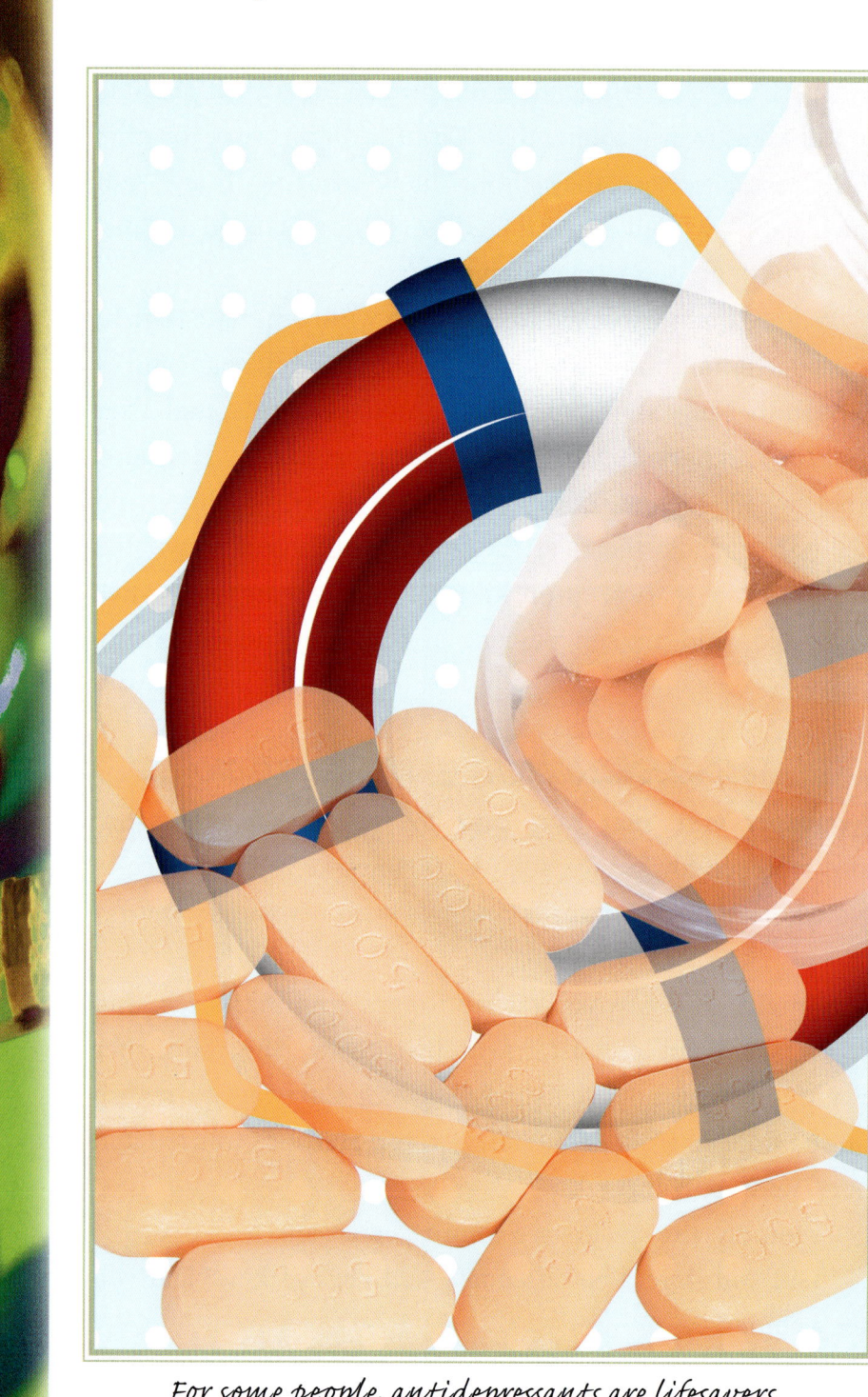

For some people, antidepressants are lifesavers.

Rebecca had just stopped taking Zoloft a week earlier, and since then she had been taking an antianxiety drug and drinking heavily. Frightened, her mother called paramedics and the police, but they could do nothing. They could not take her to the mental health emergency room because she was unwilling to go and she hadn't threatened herself or others. But just hours later, Rebecca jumped off a highway bridge and killed herself. A witness said Rebecca never hesitated. She just opened her car door, left the motor running, and jumped. Another witness, who was walking on the sidewalk below, said Rebecca never screamed.

For others, however, antidepressants prevent them from killing themselves. Gregg Phillips tried to commit suicide five times before he went on Prozac in 1998. When he doesn't take it, he says, he falls back into a black hole of depression. He lays on his bed with the blinds closed and doesn't even want to get up to go the bathroom. "Would my illness be worse off without the drug?" he said. "Definitely."

The relationship of antidepressants to violence remains difficult to pin down. Dr. Meredith Alden, the president of the Utah Psychiatric Association, says that people on antidepressants sometimes act violently because "you're already dealing with people who are prone to violent behavior . . . people who are depressed are going to be at greater risk of hurting themselves." According to Jud Staller, a child psychologist at Upstate Medical Center in Syracuse, New York, "What's puzzling and confusing about these drugs is that some people respond beautifully and dramatically to them and others respond poorly. It's such an individual thing."

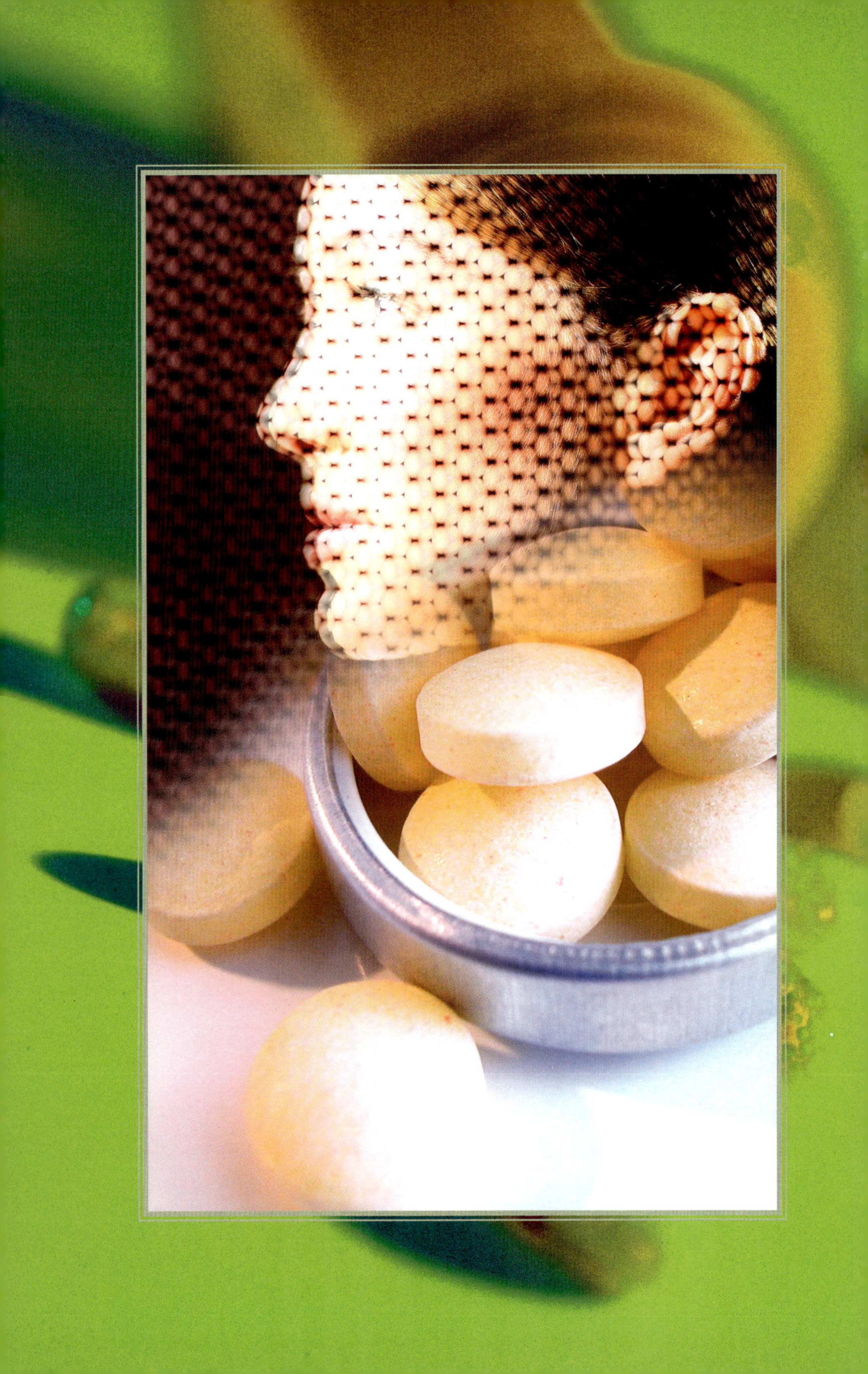

Chapter 4

Coping With Side Effects

Sometimes even psychiatrists become depressed. When a close friend of hers was dying of liver cancer, psychiatrist Nanette Gartrell began to dread going to work. She started wondering whether she was in worse shape than her patients. Her partner, also a psychiatrist, suggested an antidepressant.

Within ten days, however, Gartrell had developed insomnia, agitation, and tremors. She was unable to tell the difference between her own sadness and the drug's side effects, and she began to wonder if she would become like her father and kill herself as he had. Even though she forced herself to eat, she still lost ten pounds. When she wasn't working, she found herself curling up into a fetal position, wondering whether she should check into a hospital. After four weeks, she couldn't take it any more, so she began taking less and less of her medication. She continued to experience insomnia,

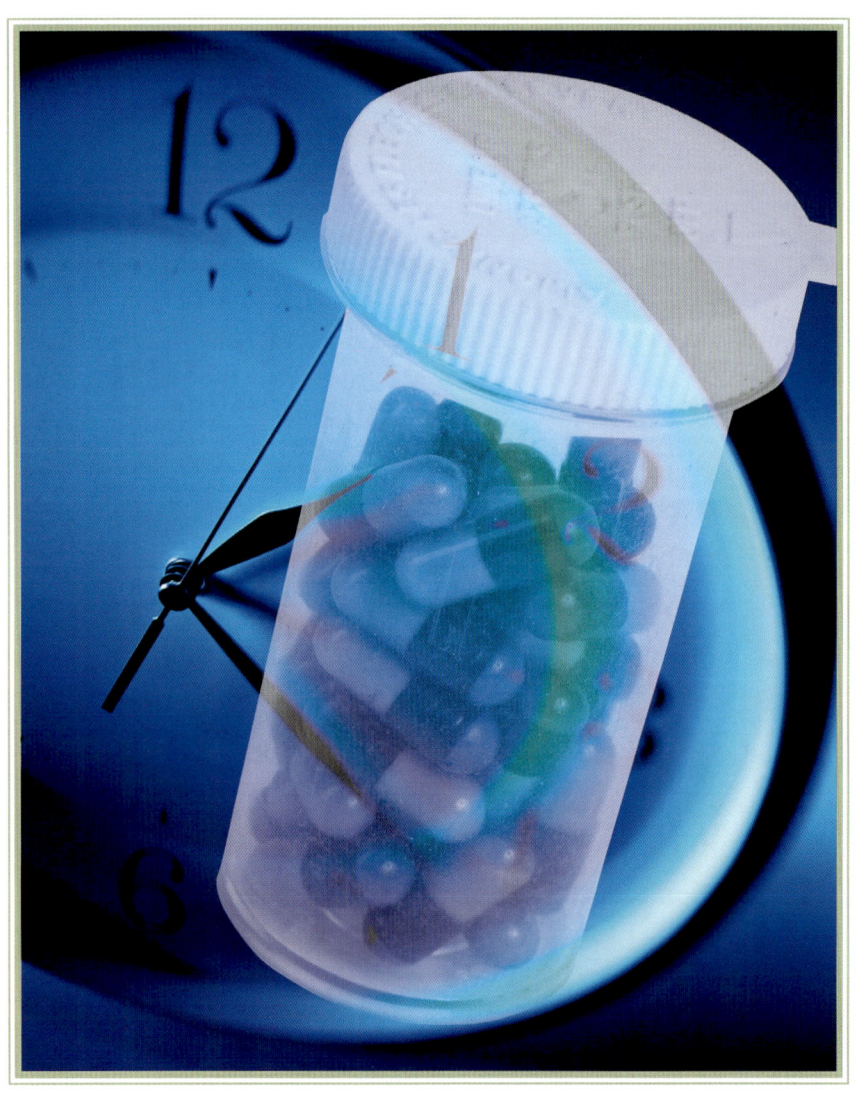

Antidepressants sometimes cause insomnia.

lack of appetite, agitation, and panic attacks for three weeks after she took her final pill, and she felt weak for a month. Luckily, her depression has never returned.

Many people take antidepressants without experiencing any side effects whatsoever. Others get them when they first start taking their medication but find they go away after a few weeks. People might also experience side effects when they change their dosage. Luckily, most of these side effects are not dangerous. Nonetheless, some who continue to experience them do what Gartrell did and discontinue their use of the drug. About 20 percent of people stop using antidepressants within six weeks, while another 10 percent stop within one year. Others, however, find ways of coping with those side effects so that they can continue to benefit from the relief the drugs give them from the symptoms of their depression.

Nausea

Nausea is one of the most common side effects of SSRIs. About 25 percent of people on SSRIs become nauseated, and about 5 percent stop taking the drug because of it. In fact, nausea is one of the major reasons people stop taking medication. It usually begins within a week of starting treatment. Sometimes it simply goes away by itself as the body becomes used to the drug.

If nausea doesn't just go away, however, there are several strategies people can use to prevent it. One would be to eat food along with the medication. While it might seem contradictory to eat food in order to prevent nausea, food can help absorb some of the drug so that it's released into the system more slowly, thus lessening its potential shock. Another technique is to drink plenty of fluids during the day, such as water or unsweetened fruit juice. More fluids in the body will dilute the drug and make it less overwhelming. An antacid might help, and so might Pepto-Bismol. Other possibilities are to switch to a pill that releases the medication more slowly into the body, or to lower the dosage.

Weight Gain

Weight gain is another common side effect of antidepressants. Sometimes this results from the body retaining fluids. Other

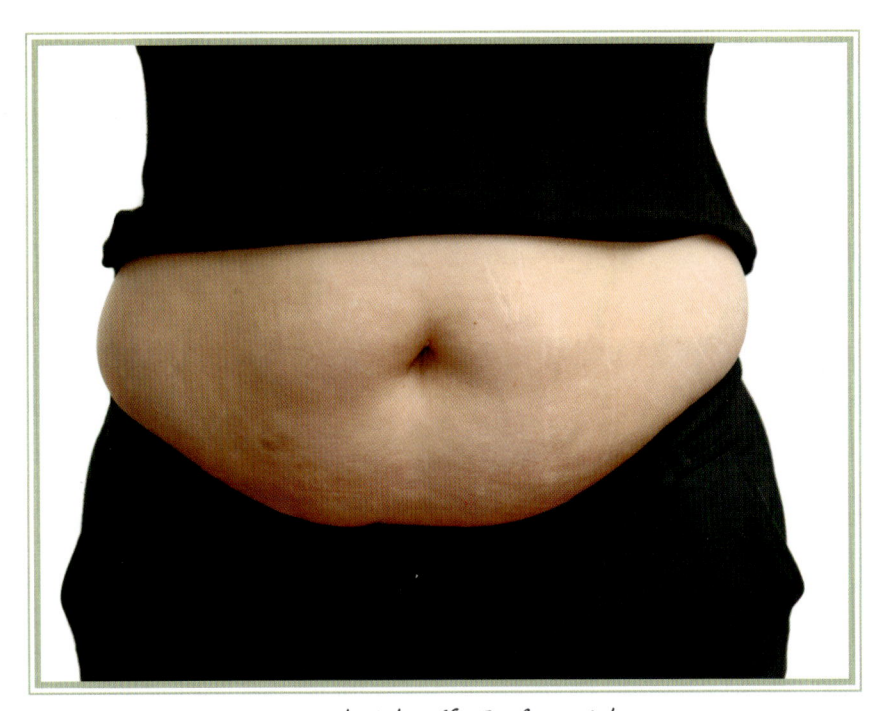

One unwanted side effect of antidepressants can be weight gain.

times it comes from a lack of physical activity. It might also come about as a simple result of feeling better and therefore being more interested in the pleasure of food and of eating. People might deal with weight gain by eating more healthy foods, like fruits, vegetables, and whole grains, and by cutting back on desserts, soft drinks, and fast food. Regular exercise could help, as well as advice from a nutritionist or dietitian. People might also talk to their doctor about changing medications. Maintaining a food diary can help people keep track of their intake and become more aware of how much they eat. Having smaller meals more often might also help because people are less likely then to eat so much at once. Also, eating more slowly may allow people to eat less. Occasionally, a

Pepto-Bismol

In the early twentieth century, when the standards for cleanliness and hygiene weren't as high as they are today, many infants suddenly contracted a disease called cholera infantum. It caused severe diarrhea, vomiting, and sometimes even death. To help these children, a doctor in upstate New York mixed together several ingredients, including pepsin and bismuth subsalicylate, and called it Mixture Cholera Infantum. Along with the pasteurization of milk and public campaigns encouraging hand washing, this mixture helped remove diarrhea as the leading cause of death in infants. In 1919, its name was changed to Pepto-Bismol.

doctor may prescribe a **psychostimulant** like Dexedrine® or Ritalin®. These drugs increase the effect of the antidepressant and help decrease weight.

Sexual Difficulty

Sexual problems are among the more difficult side effects of antidepressants for people to handle. Barbara, for example, who had been married for eighteen years, had encountered many problems in her marriage, but it was their sexual relationship, she said, that was her salvation. Unfortunately, Barbara's family had a history of depression, and as the years went on, she began experiencing symptoms herself. She got headaches, backaches, and stomachaches so bad that she would stay in bed for days at a time. At first, tricyclic antidepressants helped her, but they made her gain weight she was unable to lose. She switched to SSRIs because they were less likely to keep her overweight. These drugs, however, took away both her sexual desire and her ability to reach orgasm. Once her depression cleared, she decided not to take antidepressants at all anymore, even though she knew she risked the return of her depression.

SSRIs are more likely than tricyclics to cause sexual side effects, particularly problems with orgasm, while tricyclics are more likely to cause impotence. One way to cope with sexual side effects is to find an antidepressant that minimizes those effects while still providing relief from depression. Another is to use a drug that requires one dose a day, and to have sexual activity before that day's dosage. It's also possible to take a

Coping With Side Effects 65

second drug designed to remedy the specific sexual dysfunction that a person is experiencing.

People might discuss with their doctor the possibility of a "drug holiday" to help cope with the sexual side effects of

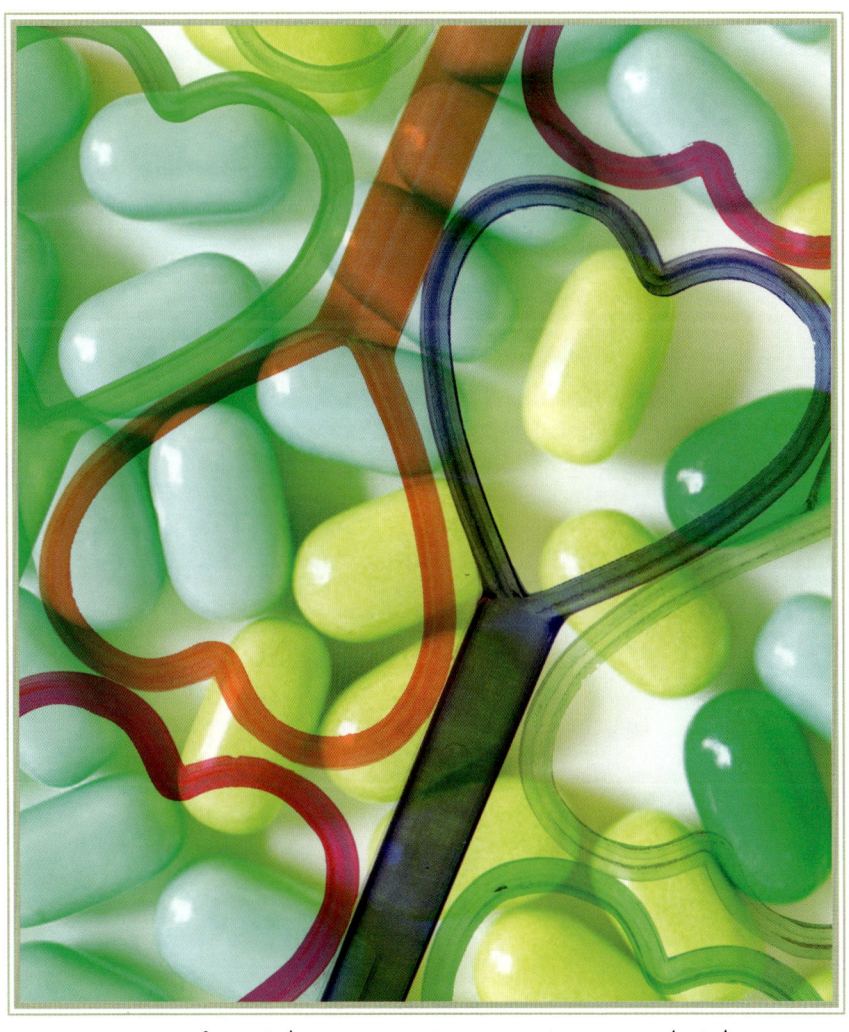

One of antidepressants' most unwanted side effects is when they negatively affect people's ability to have a romantic relationship.

antidepressants. This is something studied by Dr. Anthony Rothschild at McLean Hospital in Belmont, Massachusetts, where he worked with thirty couples. One person in each couple was taking either Prozac, Paxil, or Zoloft. On Thursday morning, they stopped taking their medicine, and they didn't take it again until Sunday at noon. Half of those taking Paxil and Zoloft saw that their sexual desire and satisfaction

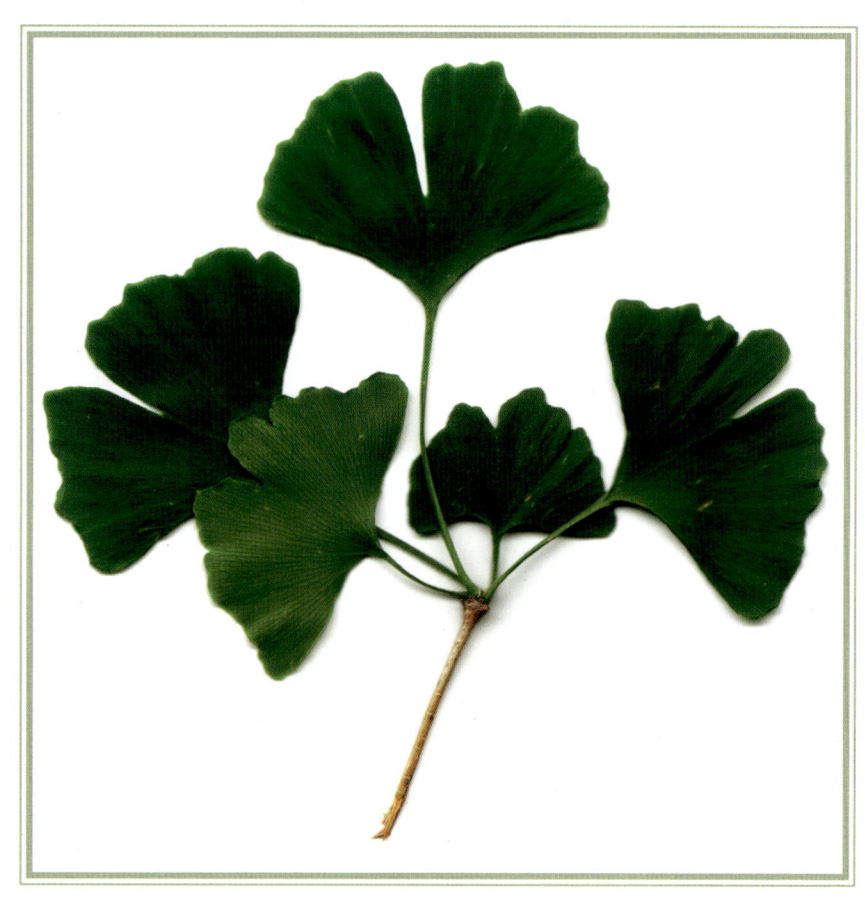

Gingko contains chemicals that support neurotransmitters and can help counteract some of antidepressants' side effects.

Gingko Biloba

The gingko is the oldest living species of tree. It's been growing on earth for somewhere between 150 and 200 million years. Chinese monks are believed to have kept it in existence because they considered its dried leaves to be a sacred herb. More than 300 studies over the past thirty years have provided clinical evidence that ginko can benefit the body in many ways. It increases blood flow to the brain and throughout the body's blood vessels, which supply blood and oxygen to the organ systems. Among other things, it regulates neurotransmitters and boosts oxygen levels in the brain, which uses 20 percent of the body's oxygen.

improved. However, only 10 percent of Prozac users received any benefit from this "holiday," probably because Prozac takes longer to leave the system than other SSRIs.

Another approach to coping with sexual problems may be to take the herb ginkgo biloba while taking an antidepressant. According to the *Journal of Sex and Marital Therapy*, sixty-three people experiencing sexual side effects from antidepressants took ginkgo extract. Ninety-one percent of the women and 76 percent of the men noted improvement in sexual functioning. While this study was too small to definitely prove ginkgo's benefits for counteracting sexual side effects, some doctors prescribe this herb to their patients.

Drowsiness, Fatigue, and Insomnia

Antidepressants can make many people drowsy and fatigued, especially during the first few weeks of treatment. Some cope with this by taking a midday nap, if possible. Mild exercise can also help. In addition, people can cope with this sleepiness by using its effects to their advantage and taking their antidepressant an hour or so before they go to bed at night.

Other people have just the opposite reaction: antidepressants keep them awake. About 20 percent of those taking SSRIs develop insomnia. In this case, they might cope by taking their drug in the morning, right after they get out of bed. They should avoid taking naps during the day because naps might make it harder to sleep at night. They might also avoid caffeine, which is a psychostimulant and will only add to their wakefulness. Regular exercise a few hours before bedtime can help people sleep, as can a relaxing bedroom routine, such as reading rather than watching television. Another possibility is for people to take a second medication to help them sleep.

Headaches and Dry Mouth

Headaches are another problem faced by people on antidepressants, especially tension and migraine headaches. Sometimes the dosage needs to be reduced as the person gets used to having the drug in her system. Healthier food and more exercise can also reduce the possibility of headaches. And, of course, aspirin or another pain reliever can also help.

Some antidepressants cause people's mouths to become dry. This generally happens when the drug interferes with

Coping With Side Effects 69

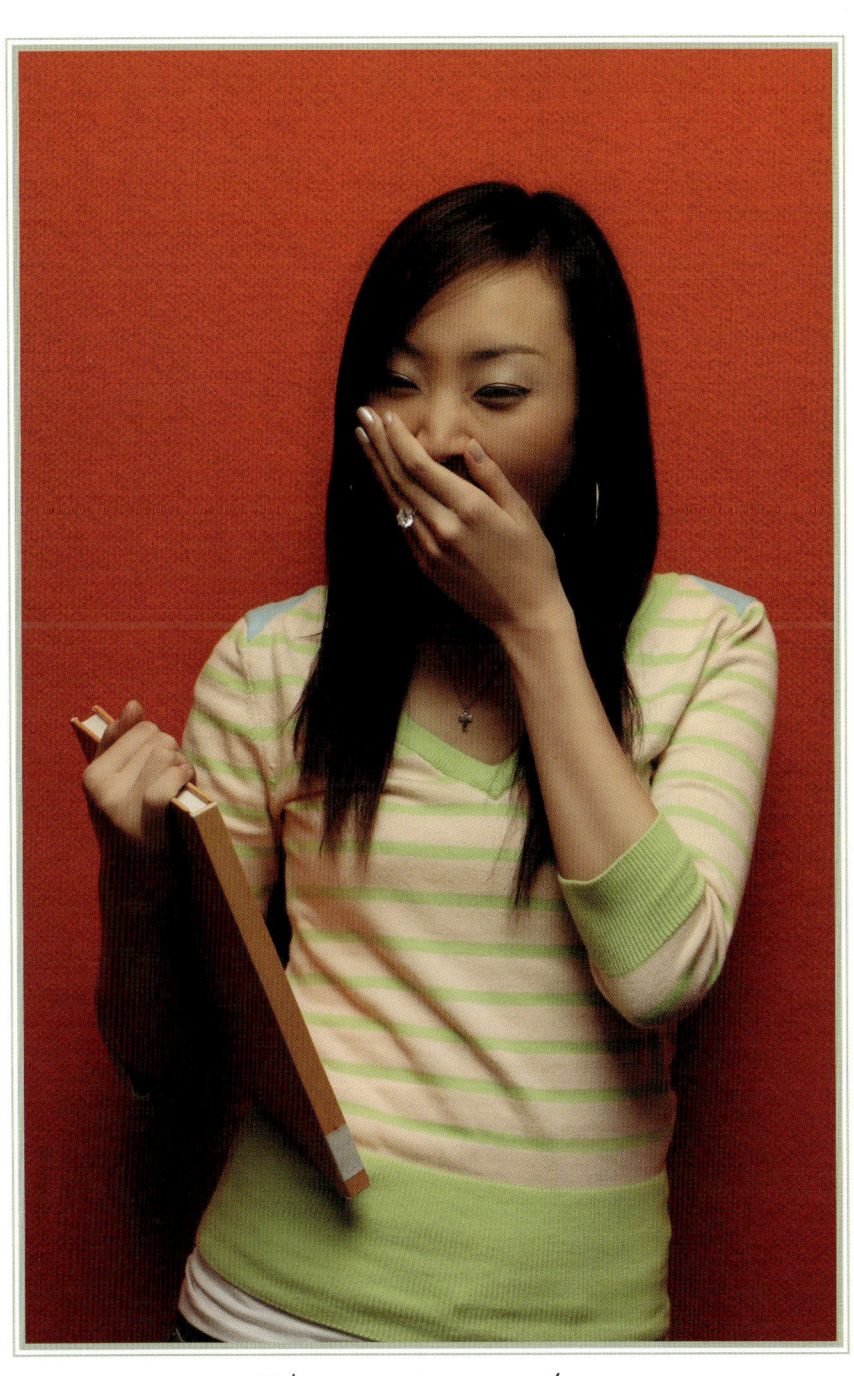

Antidepressants can make some
people feel drowsy and tired.

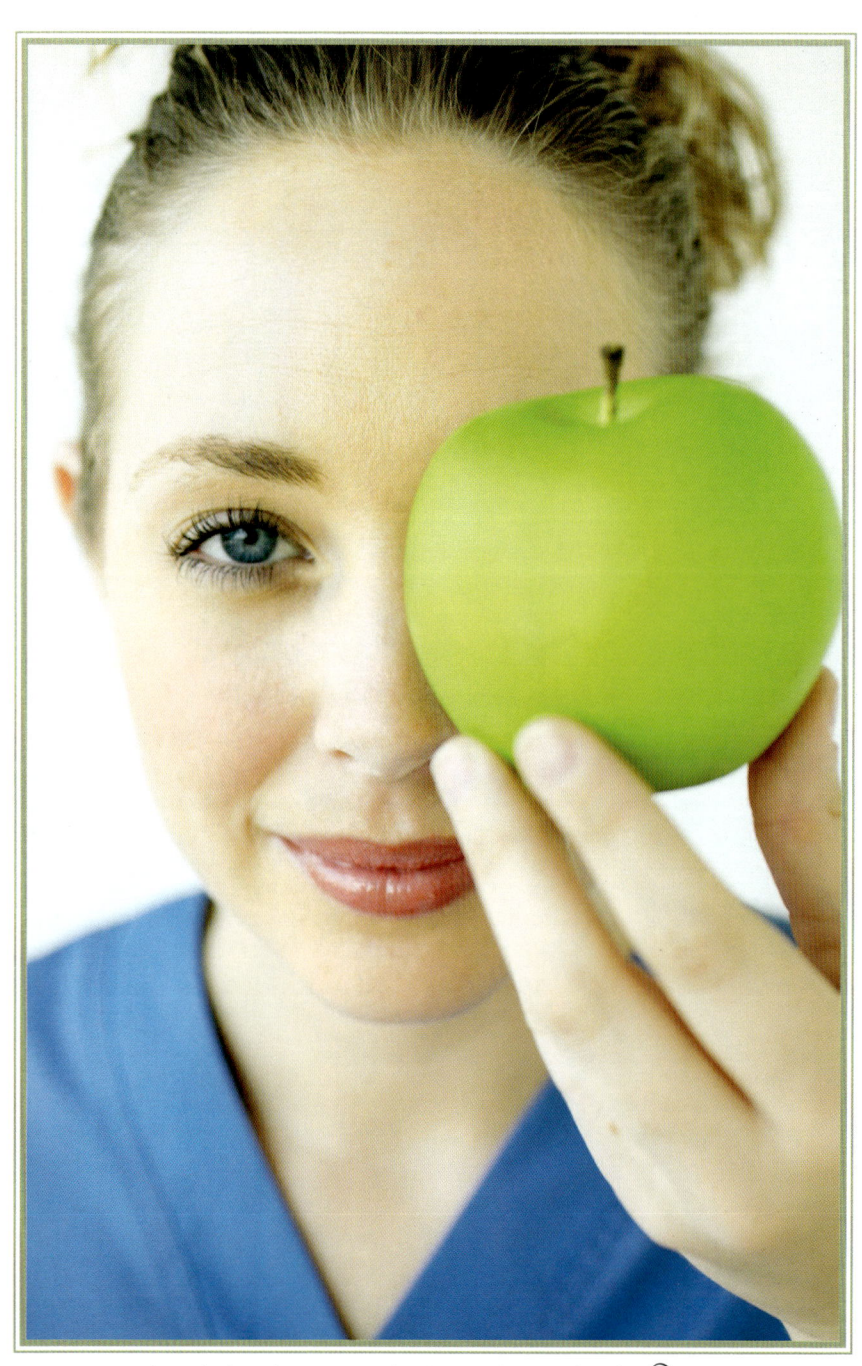

A healthy diet can help reduce the headaches an antidepressant may cause.

the production of acetylcholine, one of the body's neurotransmitters. This, in turn, can disrupt the workings of the digestive system and reduce the production of mucus and saliva. Sipping water, of course, can help this situation, as can sucking on chips of ice. Chewing sugarless gum or sucking on sugarless candy can also help people produce useful saliva. (The sugarless versions help avoid dental decay.) Also, breathing through the nose rather than the mouth can help increase the body's production of saliva. Saliva substitutes are another possibility. Good dental hygiene is also important.

Blurred Vision, Constipation, and Low Blood Pressure

Like nausea, blurred vision is an occasional side effect of antidepressants that often goes away on its own after a few weeks while the body gets used to the drug. Like dry mouth, it usually results from taking antidepressants that block the production of acetylcholine. An eye exam can rule out the possibility of something else causing this blurred vision. One way of coping with this side effect is to use special eye drops to ***alleviate*** the problem, or to discuss with a doctor the possibility of reducing the dosage.

Antidepressants that block acetylcholine may also cause constipation. People suffering from this side effect might drink more water, six to eight glasses a day, and also eat more high-fiber foods such as brans, whole grains, and fresh fruits and vegetables. Regular exercise and fiber supplements can also help. If none of this provides relief, stool softeners are another possibility.

Some antidepressants can cause low blood pressure, which can then result in dizziness. This side effect is more common in older people. One way of coping with this is for people to rise slowly when they've been sitting or squatting. Another is to use a handrail or cane. Avoiding caffeine, tobacco, and alcohol can also help, as can drinking plenty of fluids. Another way of dealing with this is to take the medication at bedtime.

Overstimulation

Antidepressants can be quite stimulating to the mind and body. While some people enjoy this increased energy, others find it distressing when they find themselves unable to be still or relax. Vigorous exercise like bicycle riding, jogging, or aerobics can help work off this excess energy. Deep breathing and muscle relaxation can also help. A medication for relaxation might prove useful in the short term. However, if this high level of energy is accompanied by racing or abnormal thoughts, it may be a sign of mood instability. In this situation, a doctor may recommend changing either the dosage or the medication.

Talk to Your Doctor!

Most doctors urge their patients to let them know about any side effects they may experience. One study showed that people who had seen their doctors fewer than three times after starting their antidepressant were more likely to stop taking

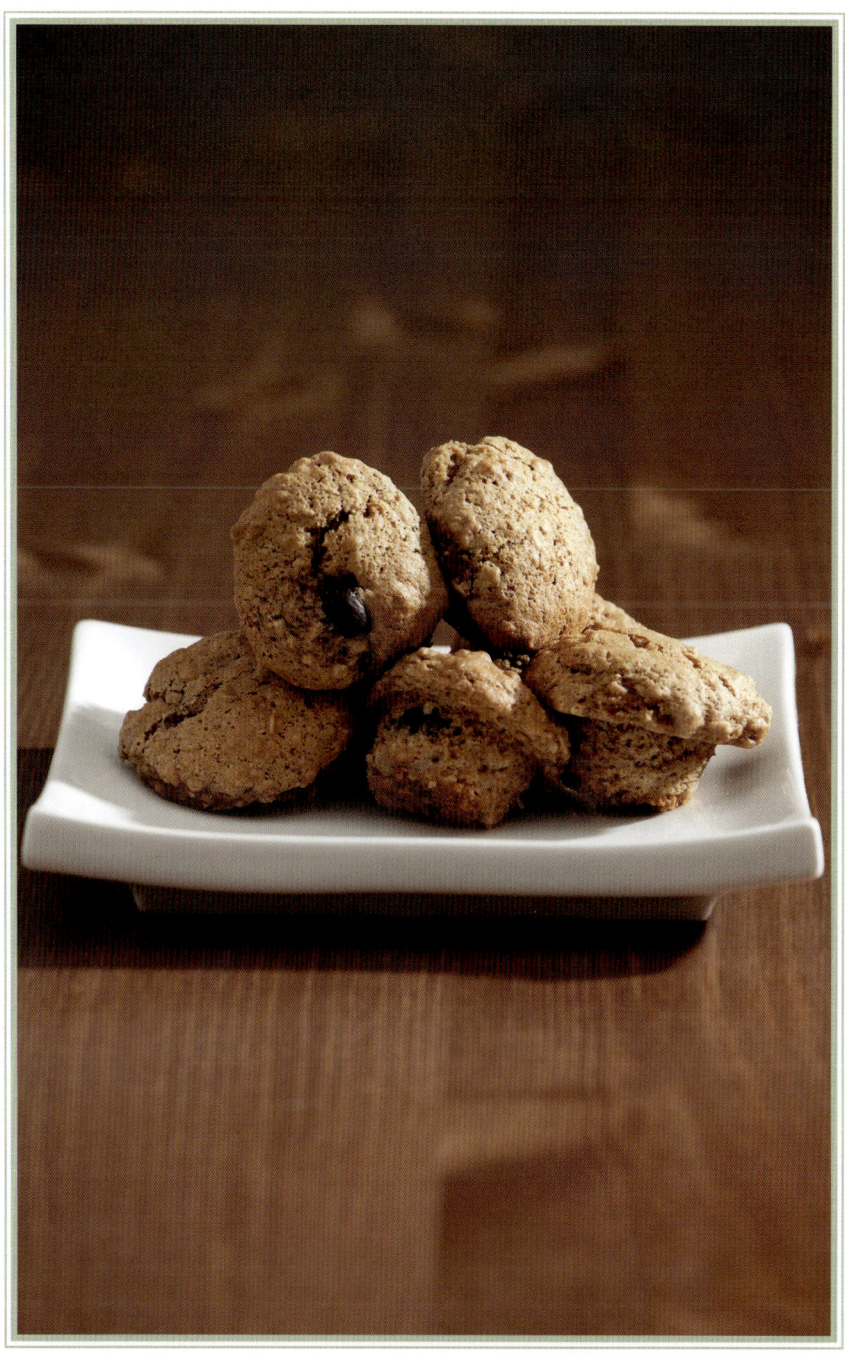

High-fiber foods like whole-grain muffins can ease the constipation sometimes caused by antidepressants.

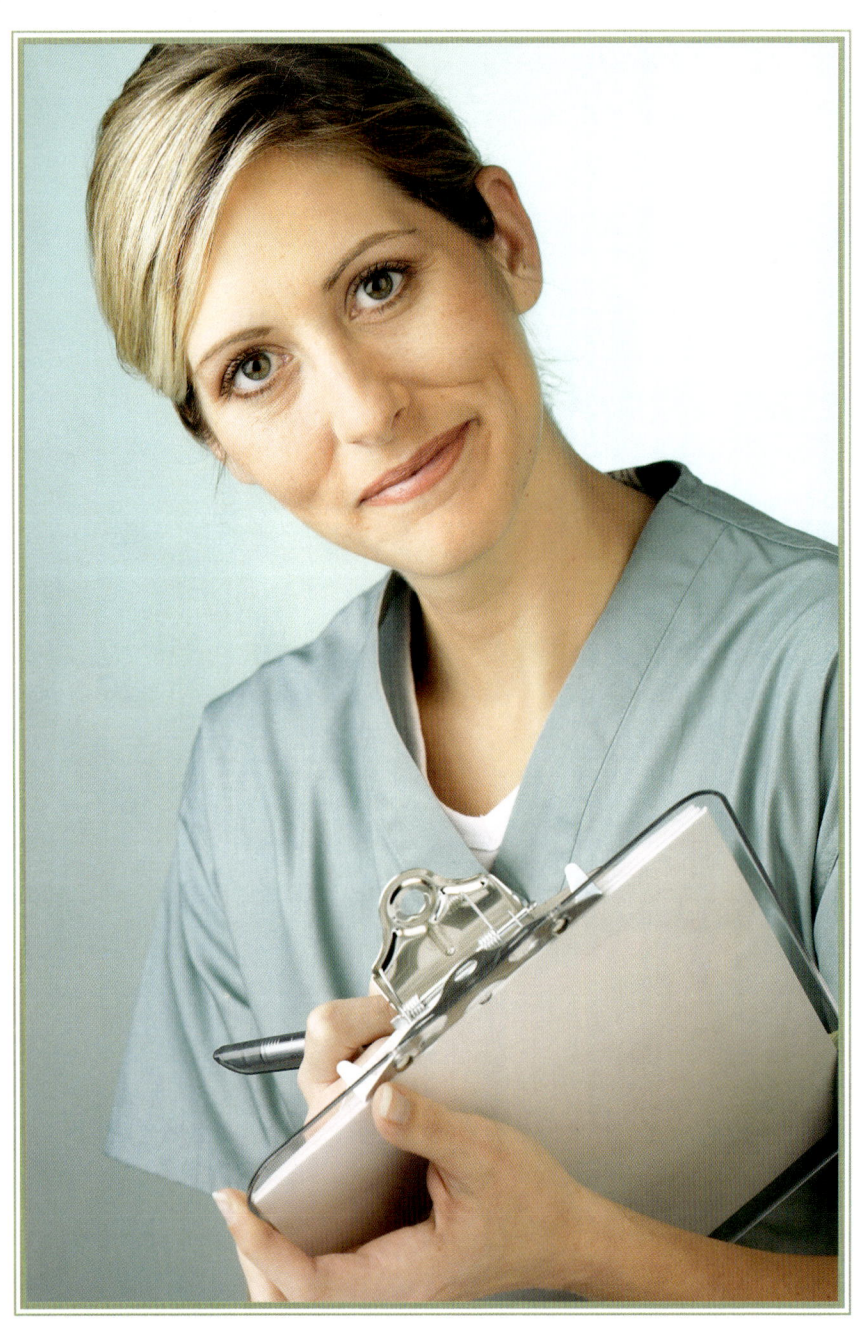

When taking an antidepressant, it is important to talk to your doctor regularly about any side effects you might experience.

it, partly because of side effects and partly because they did not clearly understand their treatment.

"These antidepressant medications are very effective for treating depression," says Harold Koenig of Duke University School of Medicine. "However, the body takes time to get used to them. They're changing your brain's biochemistry." People must remember that if one medication doesn't work, another one might.

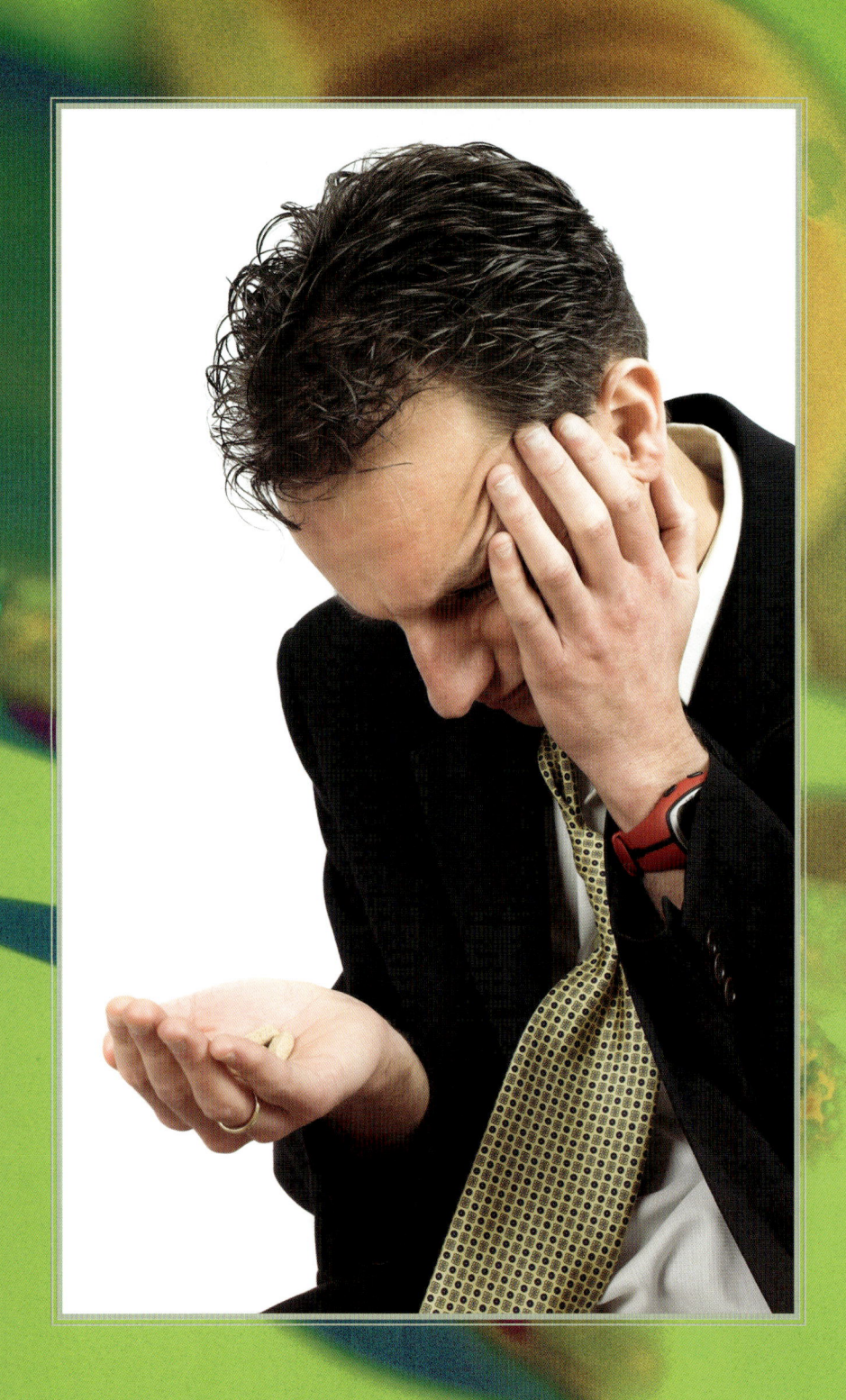

Chapter 5

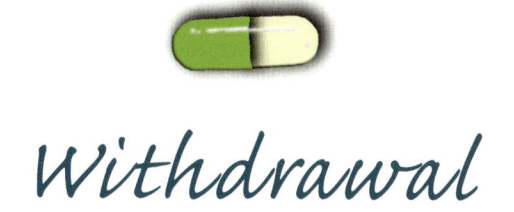

Withdrawal

Most people, at some point, no longer need to use antidepressants. Others, for whatever reason, no longer wish to take them. However, withdrawal from antidepressants can sometimes cause as many, or even more, problems as the depression it's designed to treat. While many people have no trouble at all when they stop using an antidepressant, others find it very difficult. According to Dr. Joseph Glenmullen of Harvard Medical School, "we see withdrawal symptoms that can be so severe that patients feel held hostage to the antidepressant."

For example, when Melissa Hall decided to stop taking Paxil, she found the withdrawal symptoms were just as bad as her depression had been. Even though she followed her doctor's advice and gradually reduced her dosage, she said she experienced severe dizziness, nausea, and even electric shock sensations.

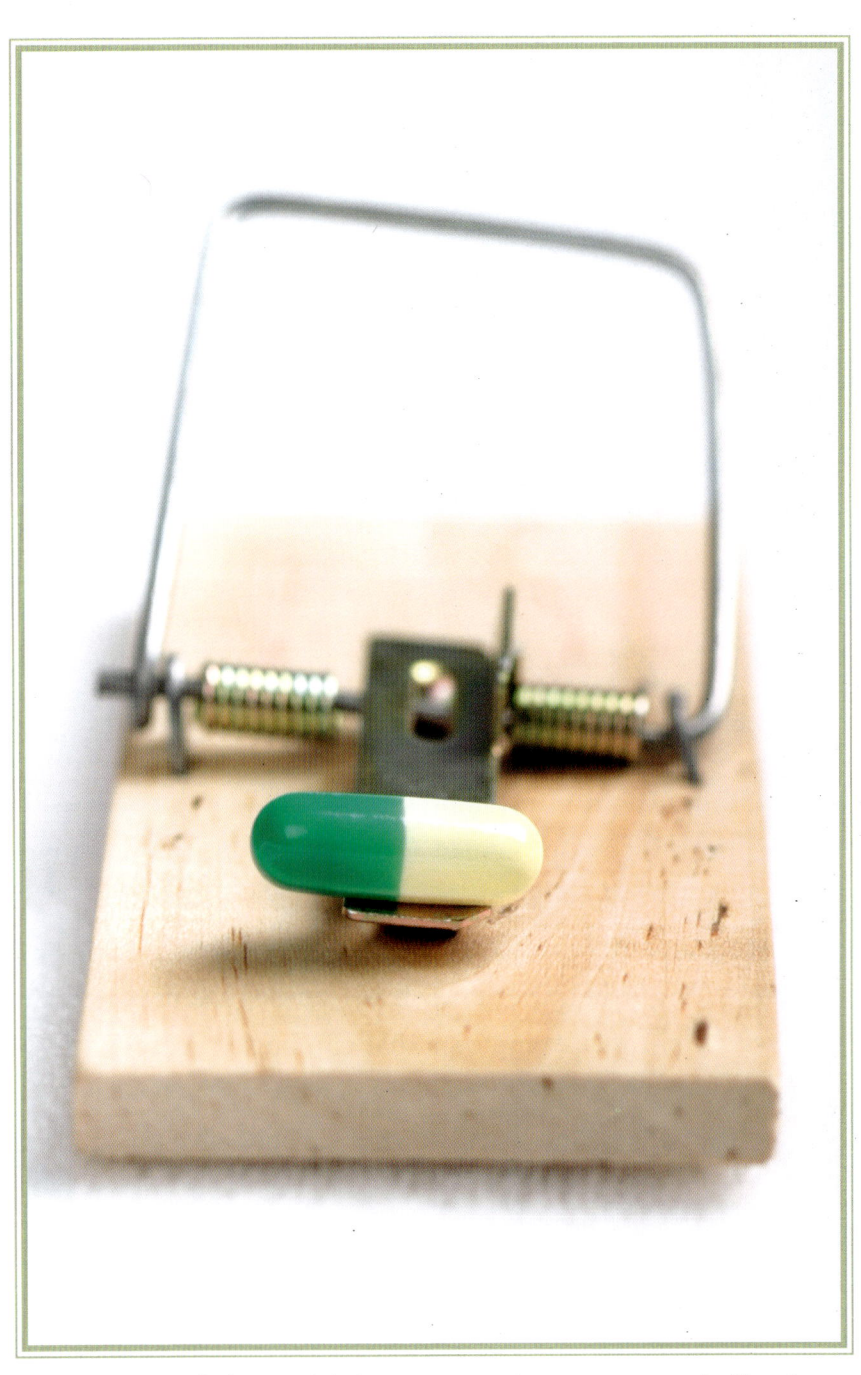

When withdrawal from an antidepressant is difficult, the drug may seem like a trap instead of a lifesaver.

"I didn't work for two months," she says on Healthyplace.com. "I just lay on my couch waiting for the dizziness and nausea and everything to go away."

Shari Loback had also trouble withdrawing from Paxil. "I was so dizzy and sick," she also reports on Healthyplace.com, "and sometimes I would get out of bed and I would just collapse because I couldn't get up." And when Kimberly Koehlinger quit taking Prozac, she found the withdrawal symptoms brutal. "You're full of rage, you're delirious, you're dizzy," she said on MSNBC.com.

Rob Robinson had trouble as well. He was a famous rock climber; he'd even been on the cover of *Climbing* magazine, and in 1998 he agreed to take part in a traveling exhibition on rock climbing. He found it stressful, however, and began having difficulty sleeping. When he talked to his doctor about it, he was prescribed Paxil. After a few weeks, he did feel calmer, and he continued taking the drug for six months. His problems with the drug didn't begin until he tried to stop taking it. He recounted his experiences in an article on money.cnn.com.

"I started having what I now know are withdrawal symptoms," he said. "They included muscle spasms, extreme sensitivity to sound, and horrible electric-shock sensations in my head." He started taking Paxil again to alleviate these symptoms. Eventually, he found a specialist who helped him get off the drug in just eighteen days. But that only brought on symptoms so severe he said he almost killed himself because of them.

As many as 50 percent of people who stop taking antidepressants suffer withdrawal symptoms. Some studies show that, after at least five weeks of treatment, 35 to 78 percent of people who either completely stop taking their antidepressant or take increasingly smaller doses will develop at least one withdrawal symptom. Some of the common **neurological** symptoms of withdrawal include dizziness, **vertigo**, lightheadedness, and difficulty walking. Some of the common physical symptoms are nausea, fatigue, headaches, and insomnia. Less commonly, people can experience shock-like sensations, parasthesia (skin crawling, burning or prickling sensations), visual disturbances, diarrhea, muscle pain, and chills. They might become agitated or irritable, or find it hard

Neurology

Neurology is a medical science that deals with the nervous system and the disorders that affect it. The first modern neurologist was Thomas Willis (1621–1675), an Englishman who first physically removed the brain from the body and described it in his 1664 book The Anatomy of the Brain. *He was also the first to call this science neurology. According to Dr. Ian Carr of the University of Manitoba, "The peculiar glory of neurology is that it deals with the part of the body which makes humankind human, the seat of sleeping and waking, the harbor of love and hate . . . the spirit which makes each of us unique, (and) the madness which sends us to the psychiatrist."*

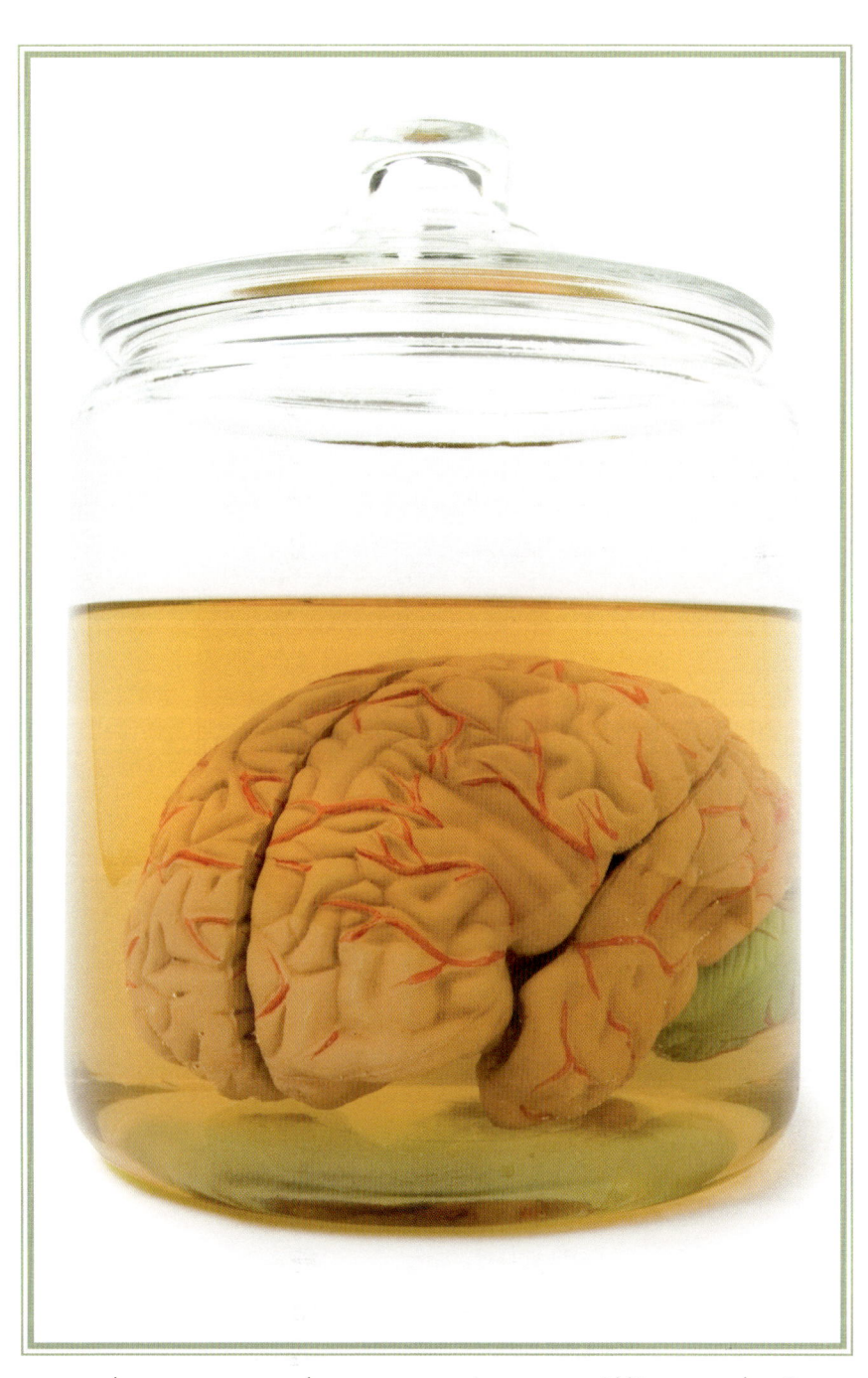

In the seventeenth century, Thomas Willis was the first to physically remove the brain for scientific study.

to concentrate. Some begin to have extremely vivid dreams. Another possible symptom is the feeling of unreality and depersonalization, as if they're watching themselves on television instead of actually living inside their own minds and their own bodies. These symptoms can appear within one to three days of the time a person stops taking the drug and could last

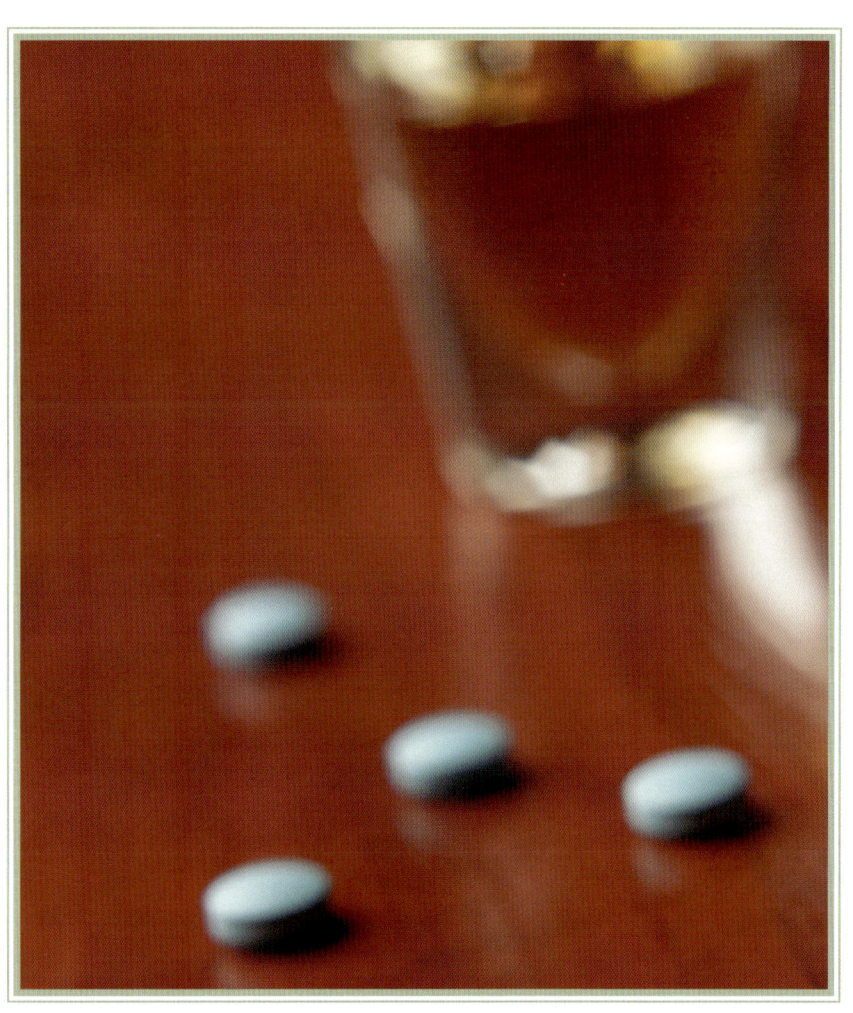

Antidepressants are not truly addictive in the same way that alcohol is.

as long as two weeks. Sometimes these symptoms can be so overwhelming that people feel they have no choice but to continue taking a drug they no longer wish to take.

Addictive or Not?

Some argue that antidepressants are not addictive. Addictive drugs, they say, cause tolerance. In other words, a user has to take more and more of the drug to get the same effect. For example, when people start drinking beer, it may take two or three beers to make them feel slightly drunk. After several years, it may take five or six beers to have that same effect. Antidepressants do not cause tolerance. People's minds do not need ever-increasing dosages to achieve the same effect.

Fred Goodwin, of George Washington University Medical School and the former head of the mental health branch of the National Institutes of Health, answers the question of whether antidepressants are addictive: "Patients ask me, 'Is this habit-forming?' I say no. But if you stop it suddenly, your body isn't going to like it very much." According to Dr. Joseph Glenmullen of Harvard Medical School and the author of *The Antidepressant Solution*, withdrawal from an antidepressant is "like throwing a car that's going sixty miles an hour into reverse. The cells were making adaptation to living with the drug twenty-four hours a day."

Variations Between Drugs

Different SSRIs affect the body in slightly different ways, and as a result, the potential for problems on withdrawal differs.

Antidepressants and Withdrawal Symptoms

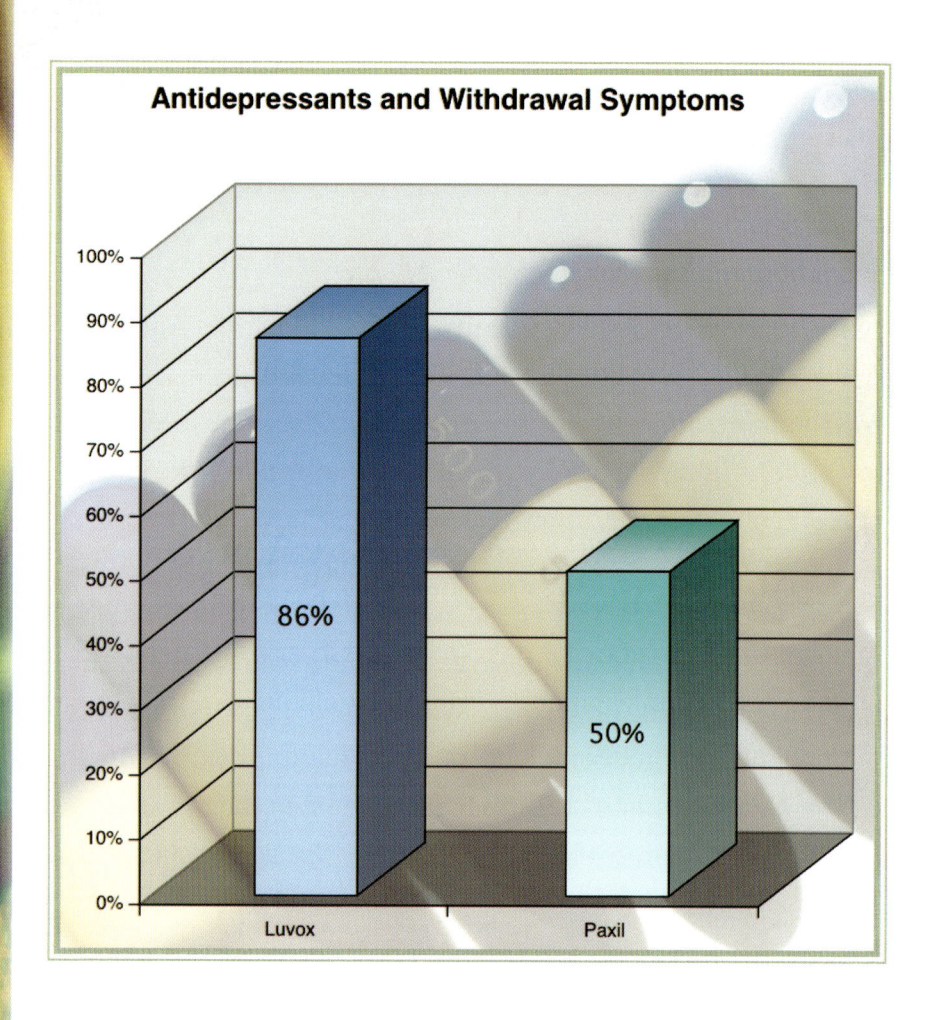

- Luvox: 86%
- Paxil: 50%

Paxil, for instance, washes out of the body quickly, and that can cause a jolt to the system of someone who has physically gotten used to it. Prozac, on the other hand, stays in the body longer and therefore is less likely to be disruptive. Dr. Robert Hedaya, the author of *The Antidepressant Survival Guide*, says that with Prozac "withdrawal symptoms take longer to hit, but that doesn't mean you won't experience them in four or five weeks."

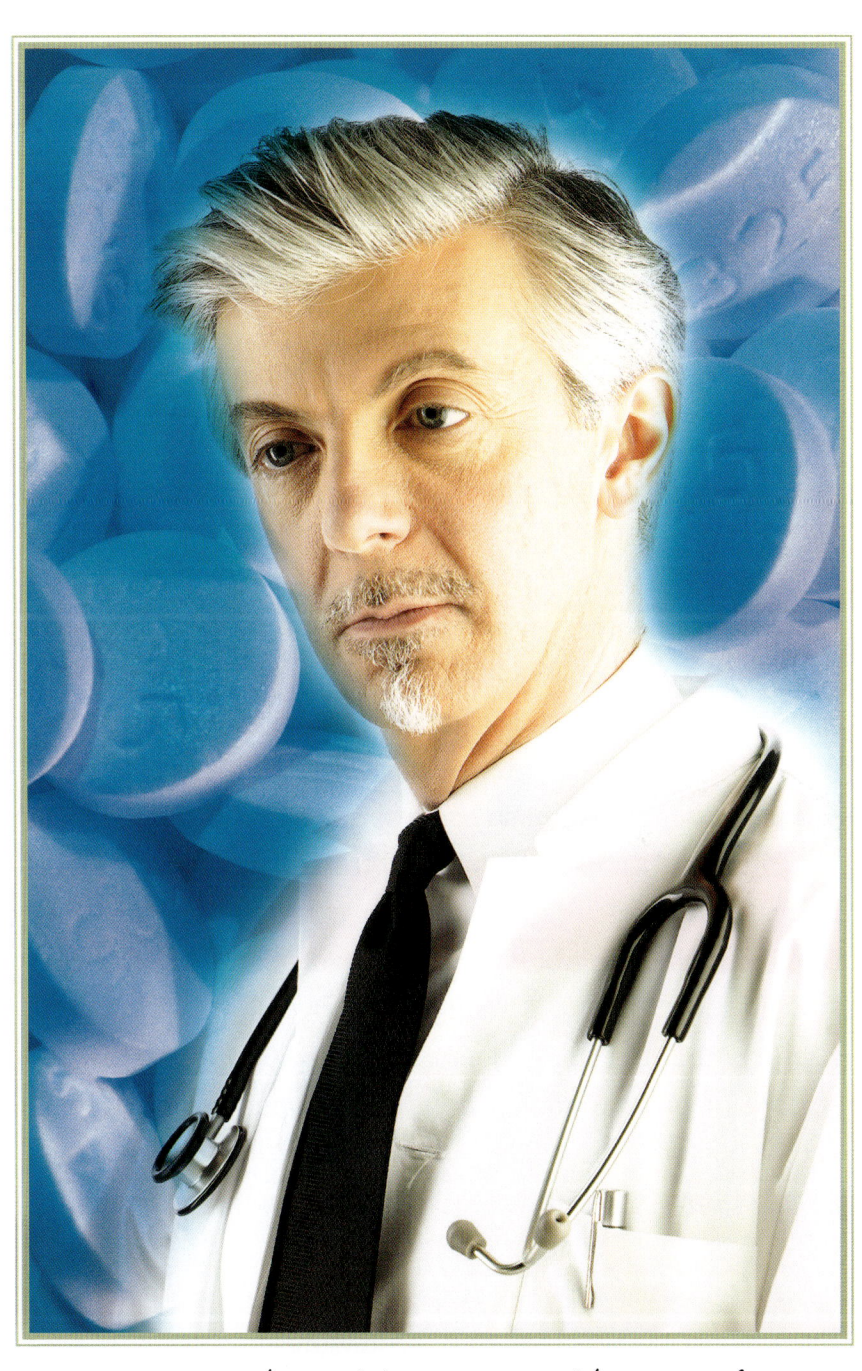

A general practitioner may not be aware of antidepressants' possible withdrawal reactions.

Withdrawal symptoms are most common in people withdrawing from Luvox. It's estimated that 86 percent of people who stop taking Luvox experience withdrawal symptoms. As many as 50 percent of people withdrawing from Paxil have difficulty as well.

Effexor, one of the newest antidepressants, is perhaps the hardest to withdraw from. Teresa Winders, an interior designer, started taking Effexor when she began having panic attacks. "I didn't feel much better," she said on nbc10.com, "and I was told, well, it takes four to five months to kick in. You've got to be patient." But when her symptoms continued to worsen, she decided to stop taking it.

"You think at the beginning, OK, I can do this," she said. "And then you start to taper off, and you think you can't because you cannot feel your hands. And you cannot feel your feet." She had muscle pain, became very nervous, and started picking at her own skin so badly she scarred herself.

"Effexor is the fastest to leave [the body], and causes the highest percentage of patients to have withdrawal," explains Dr. Glenmullen on nbc10.com. He says it can take six weeks to eight months for a person to safely come off Effexor. He also says that not many doctors are aware of that. "Seventy percent of prescriptions for antidepressants are written by family doctors," he said, and "many of them are not that aware of how bad withdrawal reactions can be."

Minimizing Withdrawal Symptoms

There are ways, however, of minimizing the possibilities of problems in withdrawing from antidepressants. One way is to

Psychotherapy

Psychotherapy is the treatment of mental and emotional disorders using psychological methods. Drug therapy, such as taking antidepressants, is a physiological method, which means it deals with the body. Psychological methods deal with the mind and with thinking. Simply defined, psychotherapy is talk. Clients talk over their problems, worries, and concerns with a trained psychotherapist, who uses her training to help the clients better understand themselves. It was first developed by Sigmund Freud during the end of the nineteenth century, and was further developed during the twentieth century by such men as Alfred Adler, Carl Jung, Albert Ellis, and Carl Rogers.

work closely with a doctor. It's not a good idea to stop taking antidepressants without medical supervision.

Slow withdrawal is best. Gradually reducing the amount of medication in your body allows the brain to adjust to the change in its chemical balance. In some cases, it may take up to a year for a person's brain and body to adjust properly.

Psychotherapy can also help. Drugs sometimes only cover up problems, but therapy can help people find the underlying causes of depression.

Exercise is another way to ease the potential difficulties of withdrawing from antidepressants. Exercise can lift people's mood, give them more energy, and improve their immune function. It can also reduce stress, anxiety, and insomnia,

88   Antidepressants and Their Side Effects

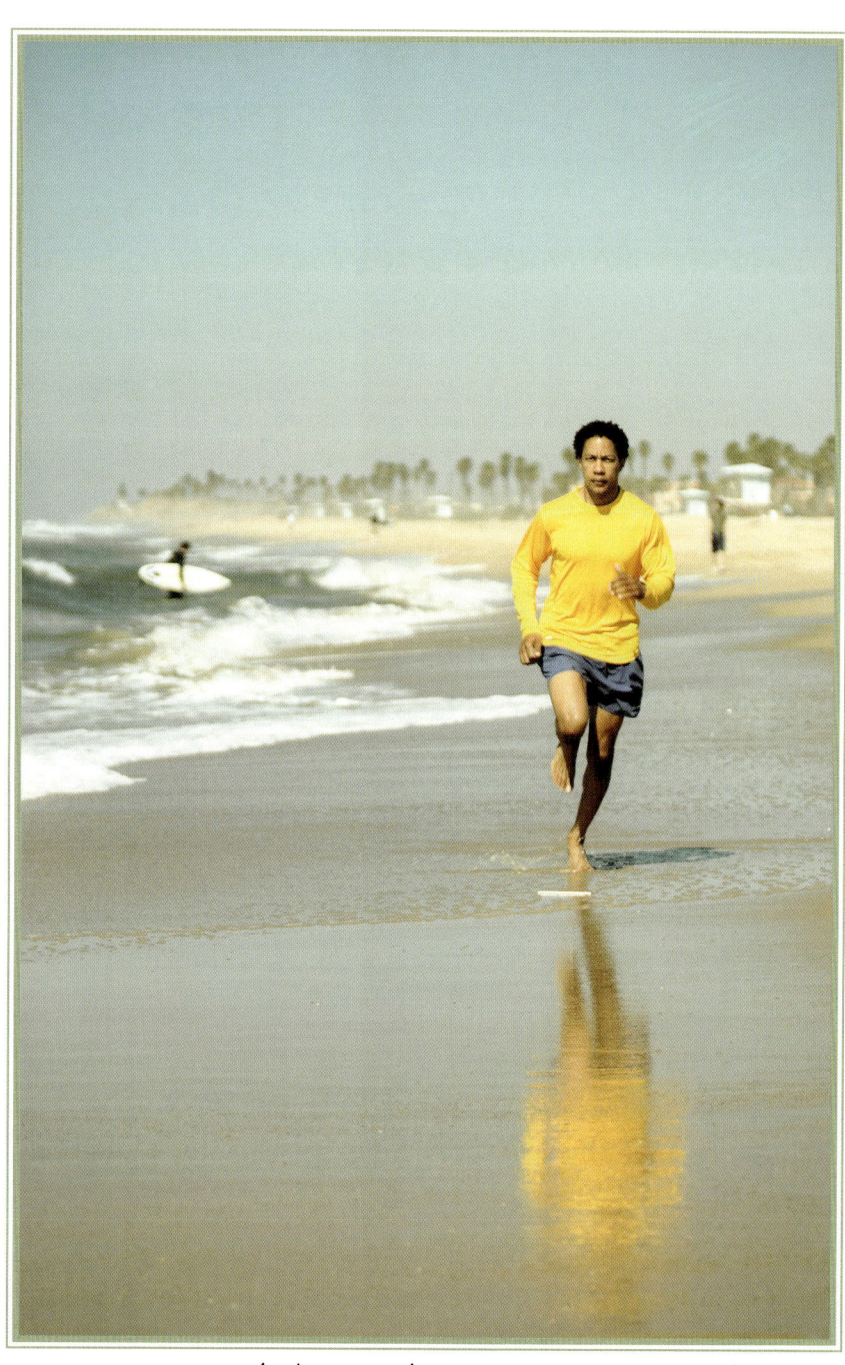

Exercise can help ease the negative reactions that withdrawing from an antidepressant may cause.

increase sex drive, and give them more self-esteem. Activities like yoga and meditation can also help.

People might also find some relief if they change their diet, at least until the withdrawal symptoms go away. Some trace many of these symptoms to a depletion of the neurotransmitter acetylcholine. Luckily, people can increase the amount of acetylcholine in their bodies by eating foods that contain it: eggs, beefsteak, liver, organ meat, spinach, soybeans, cauliflower, wheat germ, peanuts, and brewer's yeast.

Sometimes people's hormone systems interfere with withdrawal from antidepressants. According to Dr. Hedaya, "everybody should make sure they have a very thorough evaluation of their nutritional status, hormones, minerals, vitamins and immune system to enhance possibilities of reducing dosage or going off medicine." Sometimes treatable hormone imbalances or deficiencies of amino acids and minerals can sap people's energy and sexual vitality. Vitamin supplements may also help.

Finally, people shouldn't forget about their friends and family. "These are people who have been in a patient's life far longer than a therapist," says Dr. Glenmullen, "and will continue to be there long after therapy is complete."

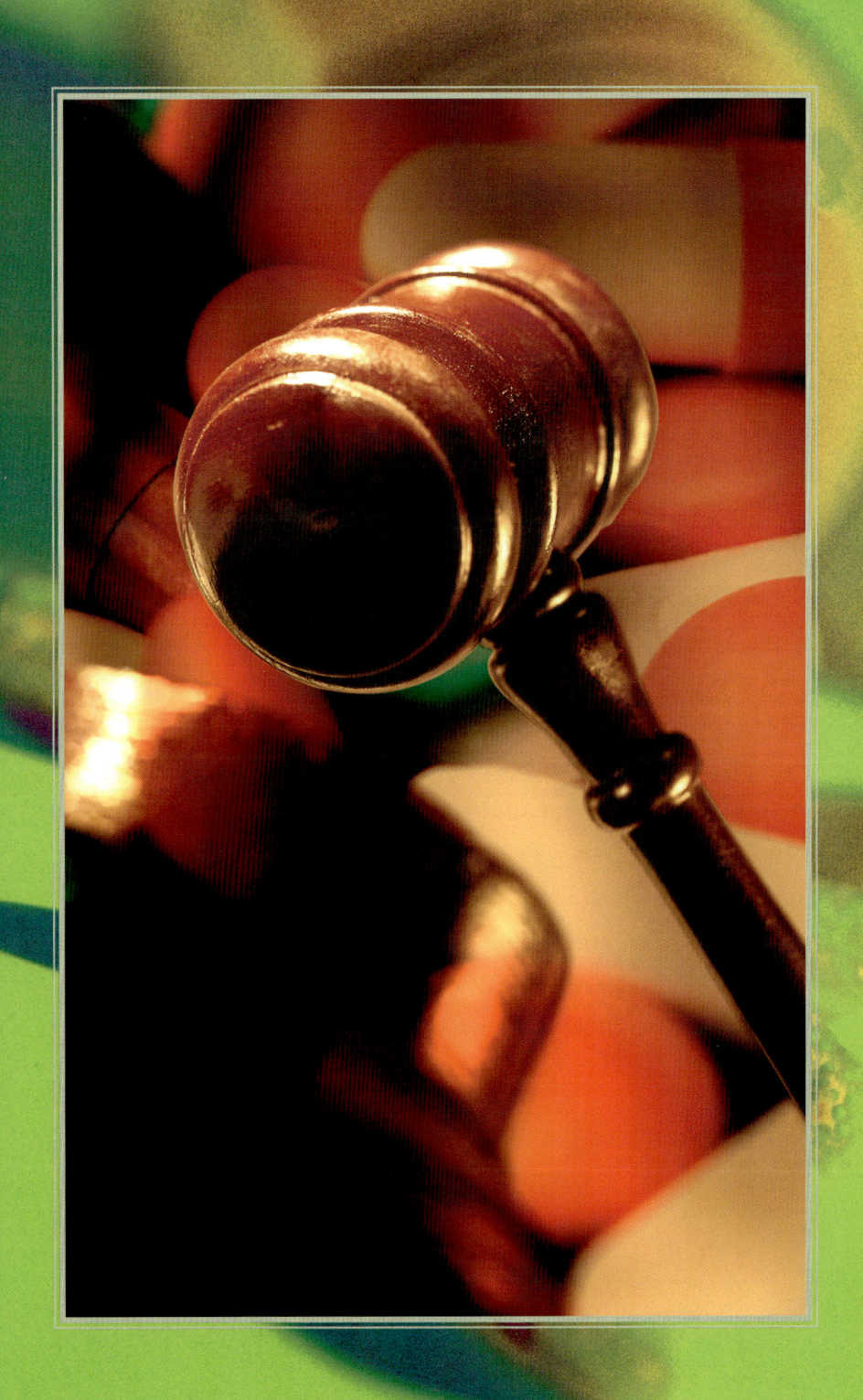

Chapter 6

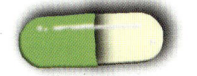

Lawsuits

Diane and Melvin Cassidy stood outside the corporate headquarters of Eli Lilly and Company in Indianapolis during the summer of 2000 and handed out fliers that said, "Lilly, how many people are maimed or dead on your drug today?"

Diane's doctor had prescribed Prozac to help her lose weight. Unfortunately, the drug gave her suicidal thoughts, which led her to overdose on a painkiller. The painkiller, in turn, caused massive bleeding in her skull and left her paralyzed on one side of her body as well as mentally impaired. Just days before the trial was to begin, Lilly settled out of court. The terms were not made public.

Hundreds of thousands of Americans claim that they have been injured by dangerous drugs and have filed lawsuits to gain compensation for the damages they say they have suffered. Since 1994, Lilly has faced more than 300 lawsuits just over Prozac. In 2002 alone, the company spent about $13 million in litigation and contingencies. Some of these lawsuits claim the FDA failed in its duty to protect people from dangerous drugs. Others argue that companies like Lilly have tried to hide the side effects of their drugs from the public. Dan Collins, a spokesperson for Lilly, says, "We do not comment on specific details regarding lawsuits." However, an investigation in 2000 by the *Indianapolis Star* showed that Lilly has paid an estimated $50 million to settle more than thirty lawsuits against Prozac out of court.

The lawsuit that could have the greatest consequences to the makers of antidepressants is the one Kimberly Witczak has brought against Pfizer, the maker of Zoloft. According to an 2005 article by David Phelps in the Minneapolis, Minnesota, *Star Tribune*, in 2003, Kimberly's husband, Tim "Woody" Witczak, began having trouble sleeping, and their family doctor prescribed Zoloft for his insomnia. Very soon after he started taking it, however, he began to experience night sweats. He had trouble with diarrhea and would become physically agitated. One day his wife was in the kitchen when he came in after having driven aimlessly around town.

"He was drenched," she said. "He'd been driving all day. He sat on the kitchen floor in a fetal position and said, 'Kim, you have to help me. My head's outside my body.'"

In early August, Kimberly left on a business trip. But one night when her husband called her on the phone, he didn't seem to be himself. He was "completely distracted," she said. "He was in a different state of mind." The next day, when she couldn't reach him either by phone or by e-mail, she asked her father to check in on him, and it was her father who found Woody hanging in the garage, dead.

Kimberly claims in her lawsuit that Pfizer didn't sufficiently warn doctors and patients about the drug's potential

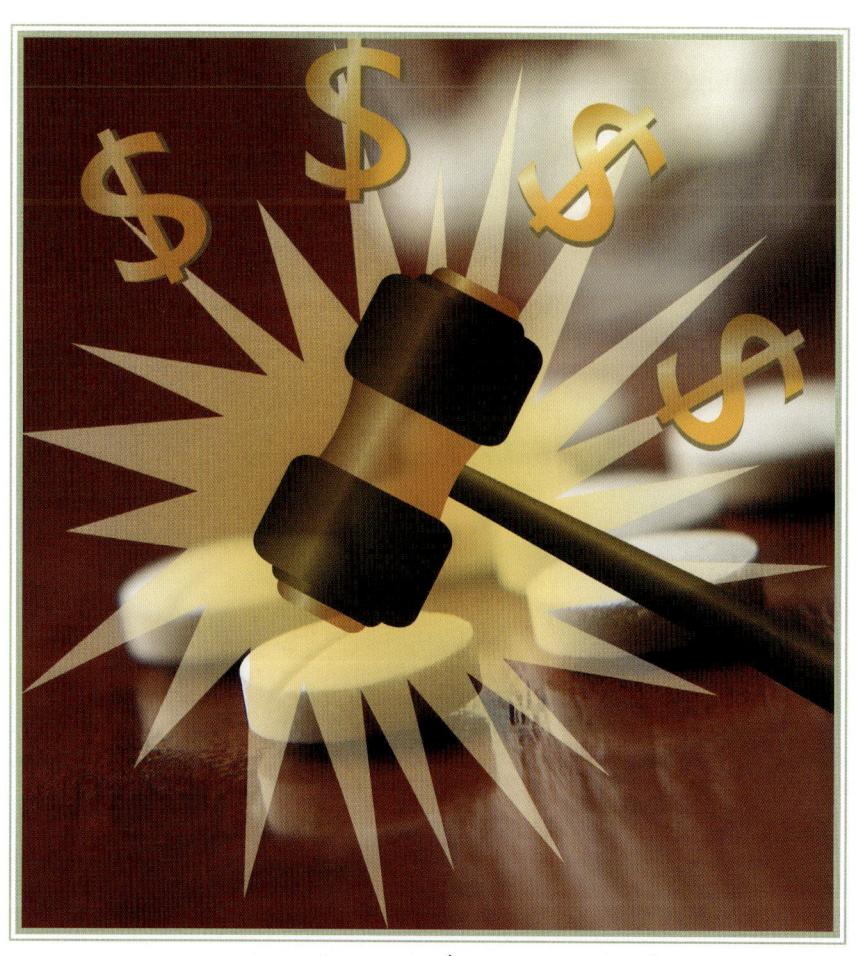

Lawsuits cost pharmaceutical companies millions of dollars.

to cause suicidal tendencies in adults. Pfizer denies this. Bryant Haskins, a representative for Pfizer, says that "There's no scientific link to Zoloft and suicidal behavior. . . . Zoloft has provided effective and life-saving treatment to millions of patients since it's been on the market."

Dr. David Healy, a British psychiatrist and the author of the book *Let Them Eat Prozac*, has a different view. "Pfizer," he said, "has been far from fully forthcoming with the FDA about the adverse reactions of Zoloft, which can lead certain vulnerable patients to become suicidal." Meanwhile, the FDA is asking pharmaceutical companies to provide it with studies of adults and suicide rates when using an antidepressant.

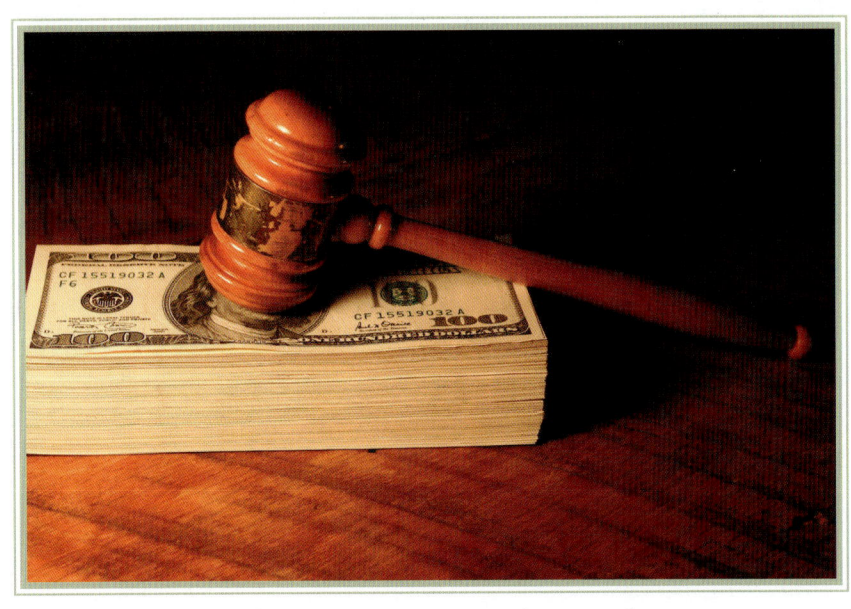

Even when companies settle out of court, they can end up spending huge amounts of money to make court cases go away.

Pfizer

Pfizer is the world's largest pharmaceutical company. It began in 1849, when Charles Pfizer and Charles Erhart decided to make chemicals that were not available in the United States. Their first product was santonin, which was used to treat intestinal worms, a common problem in nineteenth-century America. Together, Pfizer, who was a chemist, and Erhart, who was a confectioner, blended santonin with almond-toffee flavoring and shaped it into a candy cane. It was an instant success. During the Civil War, the new company supplied the Union Army with such drugs as iodine, morphine, chloroform, and camphor to help doctors treat the wounded. Pfizer began producing citric acid in 1880, and as soft drinks like Coca Cola, which used citric acid, became increasingly popular, demand soared and citric acid became Pfizer's biggest product. During World War II, it became the first company to mass-produce the antibiotic penicillin, and in the 1950s it became a major producer of all kinds of pharmaceutical drugs.

According to the FDA's Susan Cruzan, "We've just begun collecting data. It will take awhile to evaluate."

Pfizer and Lilly were not the only companies that have had to deal with lawsuits. In 2004, GlaxoSmithKline paid $2.5 million to settle a New York state lawsuit that claimed the company hid studies showing negative effects of Paxil. This fine amounted to what the company makes in a single day from the drug, which had sales of $950 million worldwide in

2004. The company was also required to post the results of its clinical tests on new drugs on the Internet.

Apparently, the editors of some of the world's leading medical journals, including the *New England Journal of Medicine*, the *Journal of the American Medical Association* (JAMA), and *Lancet*, thought this posting of clinical tests was a good idea. In an effort to help improve the safety of pharmaceutical drugs, they announced that, beginning in 2005, all drug companies that wanted to publish in their magazines had to post all their clinical trials on an online registry. According to Dr. Catherine DeAngelis, the editor in chief of JAMA, "The whole area of patient care is being compromised by not having access to all the data. We want all the studies. If you only know the positive ones, that's not going to help you."

For many people, antidepressants bring much needed relief. As Dr. Paul Goering, medical director for the psychiatry department of United Hospital in St. Paul, Minnesota, says in Phelps's article, "Do we shoot ourselves in the foot if we don't treat this catastrophic illness? If we didn't have them [antidepressants], I don't know what I'd do." On the other hand, people don't know if antidepressants will work for them, or if they'll experience side effects, until they take them for awhile.

Unfortunately, it's impossible to separate the wanted effects of an antidepressant from its unwanted ones. "All drugs have side effects, and even the safest approved drugs have side effects," says Dr. Janet Woodcock, who directs the FDA's Center for Drug Evaluation and Research. "It is very likely

Lawsuits 97

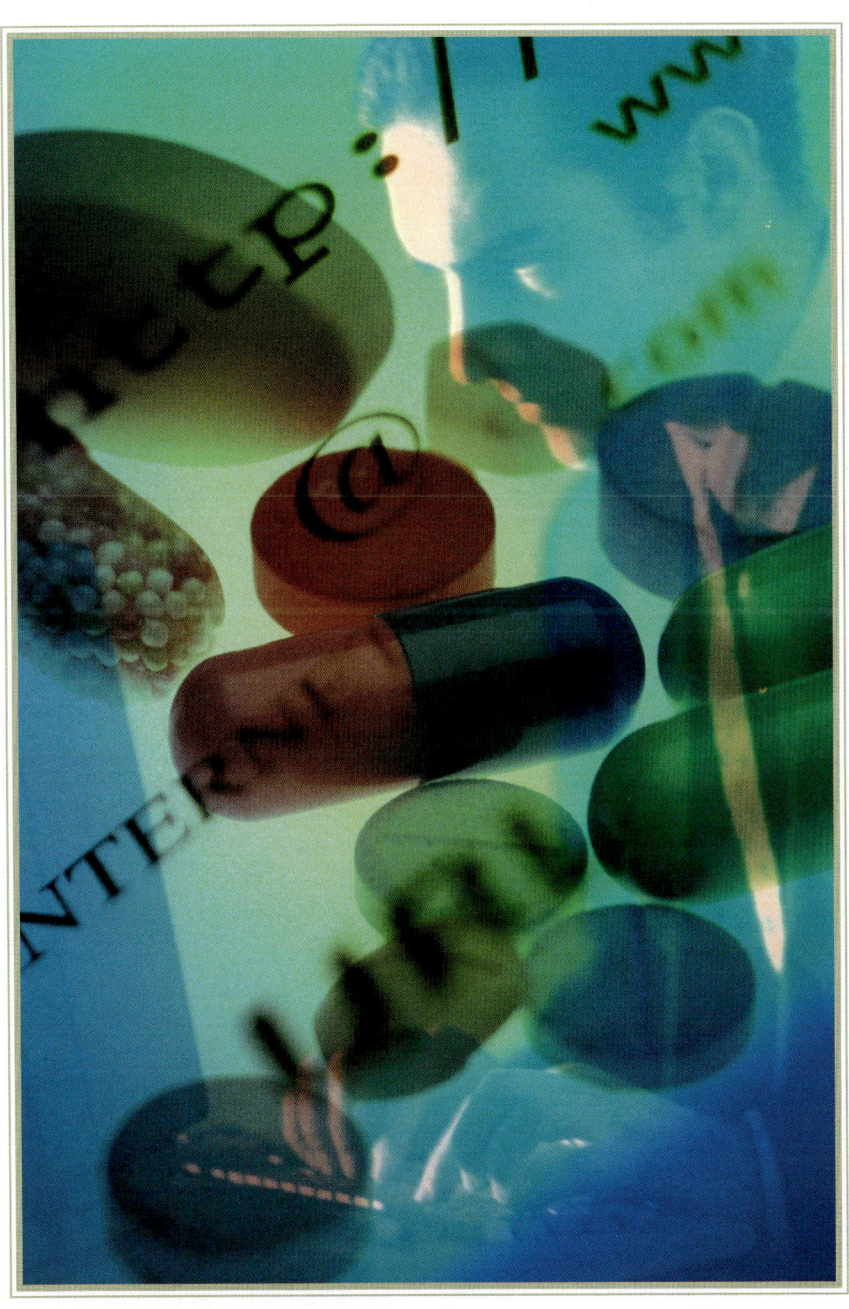

According to the terms of a settlement against GlaxoSmithKline, the pharmaceutical company must post on the Internet all results of its new drugs' clinical tests.

98   Antidepressants and Their Side Effects

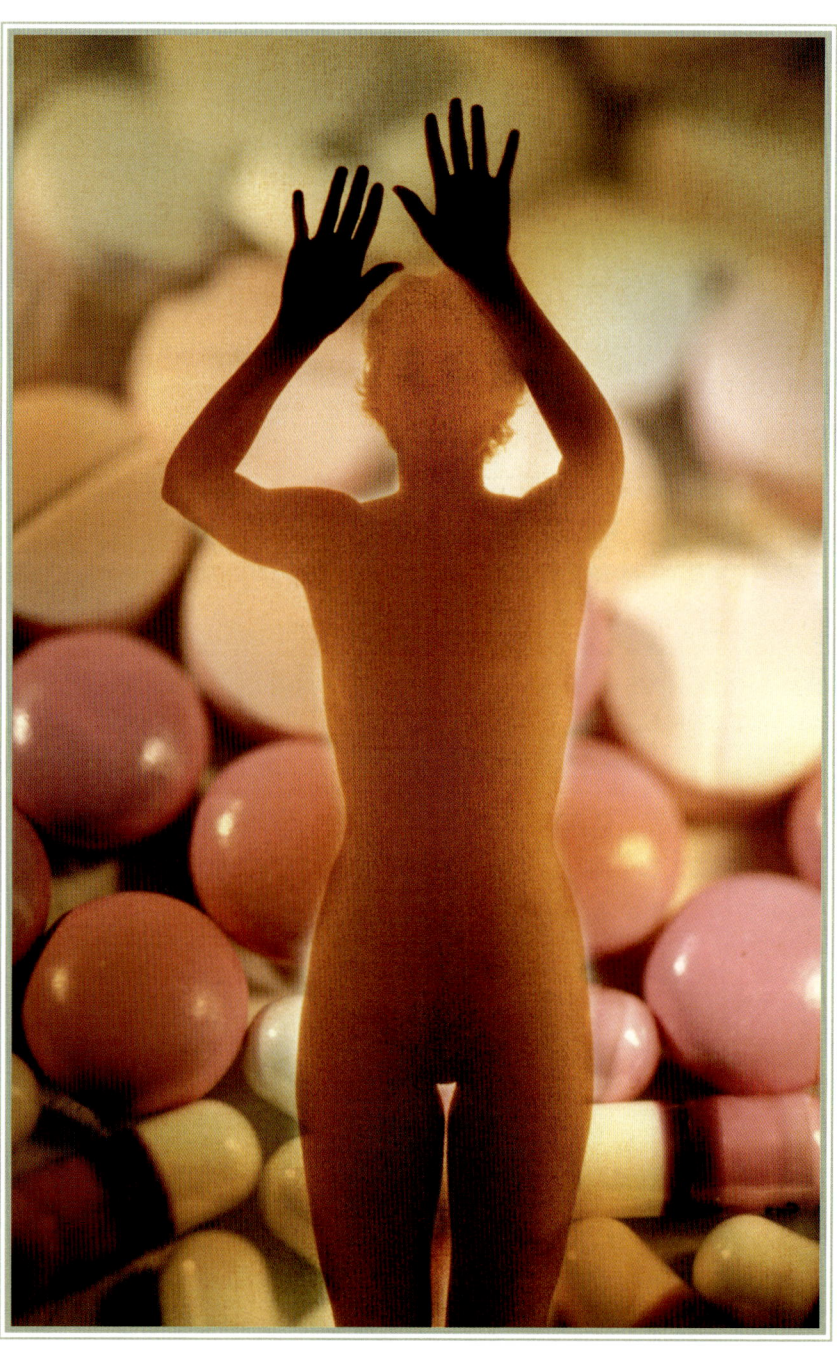

Antidepressants' effects on the human body are complicated and powerful.

that the newer classes of drugs in general are safer than older drugs, but you have to recognize that many more people are taking medicines now than used to." Dr. Joseph Glenmullen of Harvard Medical School agrees. "The problem," he says, "is that when you give these drugs to a large population, you can get lethal side effects."

Antidepressants are very powerful drugs whose workings people don't completely understand. People who decide to take them, then, should be very careful. They should learn as much as they can about these drugs and what the possible side effects might be. They should then pay close attention to what these drugs do to their bodies and their minds and report anything unusual to their doctor. In the end, it's up to each person taking them to decide whether the benefits of the drug are worth its potential risks and possible side effects.

Further Reading

Appleton, William S. *The New Antidepressants and Antianxieties*. New York: Plume, 2004.

Breggin, Peter R. *The Anti-Depressant Fact Book: What Your Doctor Won't Tell You About Prozac, Zoloft, Paxil, Celexa, and Luvox*. New York: Da Capo, 2001.

Elliot, Carl, and Tod Chambers, eds. *Prozac as a Way of Life*. Chapel Hill: University of North Carolina Press, 2004.

Glenmullen, Joseph. *Prozac Backlash*. New York: Simon and Schuster, 2000.

Monroe, Judy. *Antidepressants*. Springfield, N.J.: Enslow Publishers, 2001.

Morrison, Andrew L. *The Antidepressant Sourcebook: A User's Guide for Patients and Families*. New York: Doubleday, 2000.

Slater, Lauren. *Prozac Diary*. New York: Random House, 2002.

Turkington, Carol, and Eliot F. Kaplan. *Making the Antidepressant Decision*. New York: Contemporary, 2001.

For More Information

Antidepressants Facts, Side Effects
www.antidepressantsfacts.com

Antidepressants: Medications for Depression
www.healthyplace.com/Communities/Depression/treatment/antidepressants/index.asp

Eli Lilly and Co.
www.lilly.com

Food and Drug Administration
www.fda.gov

Peter R. Breggin and Psychiatric Drug Facts
www.breggin.com

Pfizer
www.pfizer.com

Side effects of antidepressants: Coping strategies
www.mayoclinic.com/health/antidepressants/MH00062

Side Effect Registry: Antidepressants
www.priory.com/sideover.htm

Solvay Pharmaceuticals
www.solvaypharmaceuticals-us.com

Glossary

alleviate: To make something more bearable.

anhedonia: Inability to experience pleasure.

anxiety attack: The sudden occurrence of intense fear.

attention deficit disorder: A syndrome characterized by impulsiveness, a short attention span, and often hyperactivity.

codeine: A narcotic used to suppress coughs and relieve pain.

equilibrium: A sense of balance.

hyperactive: Highly or excessively active.

inhibitions: Feelings or beliefs that prevent someone from behaving spontaneously or speaking freely.

jaundice: A condition characterized by yellowish discoloration of the whites of the eyes, skin, and mucous membranes caused by a liver dysfunction.

neurological: Concerning the brain and the nervous system.

postpartum depression: Depression that occurs shortly after childbirth.

psychostimulant: A drug having antidepressant or mood-elevating properties.

vertigo: A sensation of whirling or tilting that causes a loss of balance.

Bibliography

Abkowitz, Alyssa. "Have an antidepressant day." *Creative Loafing Atlanta*, November 18, 2004. http://atlanta.creative-loafing.com/2004-11-18/cover.html.

"Almost Half of Americans Use at Least One Prescription Drug Annual Report on Nation's Health Shows." http://www.cdc.gov/nchs/pressroom/04news/hus04.htm.

Antai-Otong, Deborah. "Antidepressant Discontinuation Syndrome." *Perspectives in Psychiatric Care* 39, no. 3 (July–September 2003).

"Antidepressant Withdrawal Can Be Worse Than Depression." http://www.thebostonchannel.com/health/4272639/detail.html.

Antidepressant Withdrawal Can Prompt Serious Side Effects. http://www.nbc10.com.

"Antidepressants and Sex." http://www.immunesupport.com/library/showarticle.cfm/ID/324/e/1/T/CFIDS_FM.

Appleton, William S. *The New Antidepressants and Antianxieties*. New York: Plume, 2004.

Berenson, Alex. "Trial Lawyers Now Take Aim at Drug Makers." *New York Times*, May 18, 2003.

Carr, Ian. "Sense, Twitch and Soul: An Essay on the History of Neurology." http://www.umanitoba.ca/faculties/medicine/history/histories/neurol.html.

Connors, Kara. "Antidepressants: Can They Turn Kids into Killers?" *Press and Sun-Bulletin* (Binghamton, New York), February 20, 2005.

"Coroner: Hartman's Wife on Drugs, Drunk." http://www.cnn.com/SHOWBIZ/TV/9806/08/brynn.hartman.drugged.

Gartrell, Nanette. "A Doctor's Own Medicine: Unpleasant Antidepressant Side Effects." http://www.healthyplace.com/Communities/Anxiety/news/antidepressant_experiences.asp.

"Getting Off Antidepressants." http://www.healthyplace.com/Communities/Depression/treatment/antidepressants/article_withdrawl.asp.

"Ginkgo Biloba." http://www.primary.net/~gic/herb/Ginko.htm.

Glenmullen, Joseph. *Prozac Backlash*. New York: Simon and Schuster, 2000.

Goode, Erica. "Antidepressants Lift Clouds, but Lose 'Miracle Drug' Label." *New York Times*, June 30, 2002.

Gorner, Peter, and Ronald Kotulak. "Antidepressants Get Black Mark: Panel Backs Warning About Prescribing Drugs to Kids." *Chicago Tribune*, September 15, 2004.

Hanners, David, and Beth Silvers. "Troubling Internet Postings Clash with Family's View of a Happy Weise." *Kansas City Star*, March 25, 2005. http://www.antidepressantsfacts.com/polite-happy.htm.

Harrison, Mimi. "Looking at the World Through Paxil-Colored Glasses." *Washington Post*, December 4, 2005.

"He Never Said Goodbye." http://www.drugawareness.org/Archives/Survivors/record0216.html.

Helms, Marissa. "Shooting Fuels Debate Over Safety of Prozac for Teens." Minnesota Public Radio, March 25, 2005. http://news.minnesota.publicradio.org/features/2005/03/25_helmsm_prozacfolo.

"History of Pepto-Bismol." http://www.pepto-bismol.com/history.shtml.

Jackson, Allison. "Drug Blamed for Wife's Death." *The Age*, May 21, 2001. http://www.antidepressantsfacts.com/DavidHawkins-Zoloft-TheAge.htm.

Jacobs, Jennifer. "Decent Into Death." *Post Standard* (Syracuse, New York), March 28, 2004.

Jarvik, Elaine. "Depressed Over Prozac." *Deseret* (Utah) *Morning News*, August 22, 2004. http://deseretnews.com/dn/view/0,1249,595085602,00.html.

Johnson, Rona. "Weise 'Always Made Me Laugh.'" *Kansas City Star*, Match 24, 2005. http://www.antidepressantsfacts.com/laugh-friends-brother.htm.

"Jury Doesn't Buy Zoloft Defense." *CBS News*, February 15, 2005. http://www.cbsnews.com/stories/2005/02/10/national/main673098.shtml.

Kaufman, Marc, and Shankar Vedantam. "Pregnant Women Warned by FDA to Avoid Paxil." *Washington Post*, December 9, 2005.

Kelley, Raina. "Health: How to Quit the Cure." *Newsweek*, August 8, 2005. http://www.msnbc.msn.com/id/8769536/site/newsweek.

Mann, Denise. "Brooke Shields' Struggle with Postpartum Depression." *WebMD Magazine*, March 24, 2005. http://www.webmd.com/content/Article/104/107292.htm.

"Medications for Treating Depression and Anxiety: Making Informed Choices." http://www.helpguide.org/mental/medications_depression.htm.

Montagne, Michael. "Patient Drug Information From Mass Media Sources." *Psychiatric Times*, May 2002. http://www.psychiatrictimes.com/massmedia.html.

O'Meara, Kelly Patricia. "Prescription Drugs May Trigger Killing." *Insight on the News*, September 23, 2002.

"The One Cent Wonder Drug." UC Berkeley Wellness Letter. http://www.berkeleywellness.com/html/fw/fwLon15Aspirin.html.

Phelps, David. "A Battle for Woody." *Star Tribune* (Minneapolis, Minnesota), June 18, 2005.

Prozac. PDRHealth Online. http://www.pdrhealth.com/drug_info/rxdrugprofiles/drugs/pro1362.shtml.

"Prozac Mania." http://www.mcmanweb.com/article-19.htm.

Reid, Brian. "Quit Paxil, and Then: Zap! Complaints Surface About Stopping Drug." *Washington Post*, August 27, 2002. http://www.namiscc.org/News/2002/Summer/PaxilWithdrawal.htm.

Schwed, Mark. "Paging Dr. Cruise." *Kansas City Star*, July 4, 2005.

"Shields Ready to Take on Depression." http://www.contactmusic.com/new/xmlfeed.nsf/mndwebpages/shields%20ready%20to%20take%20on%20depression.

"Side Effects of Antidepressants: Coping Strategies." Mayo Clinic. http://www.mayoclinic.com/health/antidepressants/MH00062.

"SSRI Discontinuation Syndrome." http://bipolar.about.com/cs/antidep/a/0207_ssridisc1.htm.

Stipp, David. "Trouble in Prozac Nation." *Fortune*, November 28, 2005. http://www.blackherbals.com/prozac_backlash_trouble_in_proza.htm.

Stollar, Christopher. "Worse Than the Disease; for Some, Antidepressants Are Not Worth the Side Effects." *Washington Times,* July 12, 2005.

"Study Discounts Link Between Antidepressants, Suicide Risk." *Grand Rapids (Michigan) Press*, January 3, 2006.

Swiatek, Jeff. "Lilly Settles Prozac Lawsuit." *Indianapolis Star*, November 30, 2002. http://www.drugawareness.org/Ribbon/Legal/record0008.html.

"Too Many Quit Taking Antidepressants Too Soon." http://www.healthyplace.com/Communities/Depression/treatment/antidepressants/article_staying_on.asp.

"Tricyclic antidepressants." http://www.mayoclinic.com/health/antidepressants/MH00071.

Vedantam, Shankar. "Antidepressant Use by U.S. Adults Soars." *Washington Post*, December 3, 2004. http://www.washingtonpost.com/wp-dyn/articles/A29751-2004Dec2.html.

Waters, Rob. "My Antidepressant Made Me Do It!" *Salon.* http://www.salon.com/health/feature/1999/07/19/zoloft/print.html.

"Wellbutrin." http://www.pdrhealth.com/drug_info/rxdrugprofiles/drugs/wel1488.shtml.

"White Willow." *Encyclopedia of Alternative Medicine* http://health.enotes.com/alternative-medicine-encyclopedia/white-willow/print.

Whitney, Tom. "That's Me, a Marine, a Murderer of Civilians." *San Francisco Bay View*, March 13, 2005. http://www.sfbayview.com/030905/amarine030905.shtml.

Williams, Daniel. "Bitter Pills." *Time International*, November 21, 2005.

Young, Emma. "Prozac Triggers Increase in Aggression in Mice." *New Scientist*, November 12, 2001. http://www.newscientist.com/article.ns?id=dn1553.

Index

abnormal dreams 18
abnormal ejaculation 18, 38
abnormal vision 18
adult violence 47–49
agitation 40, 59, 61, 92
Alliance for Human Research Protection 47
anhedonia 12
anxiety 18, 21, 36, 52
aspirin 14, 16, 17, 68
attention deficit disorder 25
axon 14

bipolar disorder 52
black box warning 27
blurred vision 18, 71

Celexa (citalopram) 10, 36, 46
cholesterol 31, 32
Clozaril (clozapine) 52
codeine 11
Columbine High School shootings 43–44
constipation 40, 71
coping with side effects 27–28, 30–31

Department of Health and Human Services 35
Dexedrine 64
diarrhea 18, 80, 92
diminished sex drive 18

dizziness 18, 36, 40, 72, 79, 80
dopamine 40
drowsiness 18, 68
dry mouth 18, 40, 68, 71

Effexor 46, 48, 86
Elavil (amitriptyline) 17
electric-shock sensations 77, 79, 80
Eli Lilly and Company 46, 47, 91, 92, 95

fatigue 68, 80
flu-like symptoms 18
flushing 18
Food and Drug Administration (FDA) 27, 28, 46, 50, 92, 94, 95, 96

gingko biloba 67
GlaxoSmithKline 95, 97

Haldol (haloperidol) 52
Hartman, Phil 48
head banging 32
headaches 18, 40, 64, 68, 80
hemorrhages 18
high blood pressure 18, 19, 31
hopelessness 12
hyperactivity 26

imipramine 18
impotence 18, 38
insomnia 12, 18, 59, 60, 68, 80, 92
iproniazid 17, 18, 19
itching 18

jaundice 18

lawsuits 91–96, 99
Lexapro (escitalopram) 10, 38
Librium (chlordiazepoxide) 52
lithium 52
long-term use of antidepressants 31
loss of appetite 12, 18, 59, 60, 61
low blood pressure 72
Luvox (fluvoxamine) 10, 44, 86

mania 44
murder 41, 46
muscle spasms 79

nausea 18, 40, 41, 61, 79, 80
nervousness 18
neurons 13, 14
neurotransmitters 14, 15, 17, 40, 71
norepinephrine 40
non-SSRI antidepressants 41

panic attacks 61, 86
Paxil (paroxetine) 10, 28, 30, 31, 32, 33, 35, 36, 50, 66, 77, 79, 84, 86, 95
personality disorder 36
Pfizer Pharmaceuticals 92, 93, 94, 95
Physician's Desk Reference (PDR) 18, 20, 44
postpartum depression 9–10, 11, 20, 21
Prozac (fluoxetine) 10, 18, 23, 27, 28, 39, 46, 47, 57, 66, 67, 79, 84, 91, 92
psychostimulant 64, 68
psychotherapy 87
psychotropic drugs 52

Remeron 48
Ritalin 64

Saturday Night Live 47
schizophrenia 52
seizures 40
self-mutilation 35
serotonin 13, 15
serotonin reuptake inhibitors (SSRIs) 10–11, 17, 18, 20, 27, 28, 30, 40, 47, 61, 64, 67, 68, 83
Serzone 41
sexual side effects 18, 38–41, 64–67
Shields, Brooke 9–10, 11, 21
sinusitis 18
skin rash 18, 40
sleep disturbances 40
sleepiness 18
Solvay Pharmaceuticals Inc. 44
sore throat 18
sound sensitivity 79
stomach bleeding 17
suicide 26, 27, 34, 35, 41, 43–44, 47, 48, 55, 57, 59, 91, 93, 94
Surmontil (trimipramine) 17
sweating 18, 40, 92
synapse 14, 15

teen violence 44–47
Thorazine (chlorpromazine) 52
thoughts of death 12
Tofranil (imipramine) 17
tremors 20, 30, 40, 59
tricyclics 17, 40, 64
tuberculosis 18

upset stomach 20

vertigo 80
vomiting 20

weakness 20, 79
weight gain 30, 36, 62, 64
Wellbutrin (bupropion) 36, 40

withdrawal 77, 79–80, 82–84, 86–87, 89

Yates, Andrea 48
yawning 20

Zoloft (sertraline) 10, 21, 26, 41, 48, 49, 50, 57, 66, 92, 94

Picture Credits

Benjamin Stewart: pp. 56, 60, 65, 84, 90
iStockphotos: pp. 62, 93
    Andrew Taylor: p. 78
    Bonnie Jacobs: p. 42
    Charlotte Erpenbeck: p. 66
    Duncan Walker: p. 26
    Karen Towne: p. 54
    Kenneth C. Zirkel: p. 81
    Nathan Watkins: p. 31
    Peter Chen: p. 69
    Roberta Osborne: p. 45
    Sharon Dominick: p. 33
    Simon van den Berg: p. 76
    Stefan Klein: pp. 51, 94
    Valentin Casarsa: p. 49
Jupiter Images: pp. 8, 13, 15, 16, 19, 20, 22, 24, 34, 37, 39, 53, 58, 70, 73, 74, 82, 85, 88, 97, 98
Moono.com: p. 11

Biographies

Author

Craig Russell teaches writing at Broome Community College in Binghamton, New York. He has written several nonfiction books for young adults.

Consultant

Andrew M. Kleiman, M.D., received a Bachelor of Arts degree in philosophy from the University of Michigan, and earned his medical degree from Tulane University School of Medicine. Dr. Kleiman completed his internship, residency in psychiatry, and fellowship in forensic psychiatry at New York University and Bellevue Hospital. He is currently in private practice in Manhattan, specializing in psychopharmacology, psychotherapy, and forensic psychiatry. He also teaches clinical psychology at the New York University School of Medicine.